Tales of the Exam Room Volume 3: **Medical Stories While Incarcerated**

This is a work of fiction. Unless otherwise stated – all names, characters, businesses, places, events, locales, and incidents in this book are the product of either the author's imagination or are used in a fictitious manner. Any resemblance to actual persons, living or dead, or actual events is purely coincidental.

ISBN: 978-1-954814-02-8 (Paperback)

ISBN: 978-1-954814-03-5 (EBook)

Purple Background Cover

Second Edition 2021.

Credits:

Book Cover and Formatting by farhanshahid101

Obsidian Wolf Publishing

PO Box 1086 Salem, UT 84653

Contents

Correctional Medicine

The United States has, by far, one of the highest rates of incarcerations in the world. As of 2016 – 655 inmates per 100,000 are found within the jails and prisons of America. But other countries around the world are also experiencing an ncrease in the number of individuals incarcerated. Many different countries have tried different things to curb incarceration rates – some work, and some do not.

Each country has specific and unique ways to handle the medical needs required for inmates. This need may be overlooked o· misunderstood when dealing with cost, workforce, funding, and many other areas of correctional responsibilities.

Additionally, millions of individuals have been freed from jails and prisons that are being monitored on probation or parcle. This also adds to the responsibilities of the government, cities, towns, and communities. For those younger than 18 – there are often detention centers.

Correctional Med cine is challenging and unique. Inmates can be difficult to treat for several reasons, including risk factors, past medical histories, unique circumstances, unique mental health problems, difficulty following directions, homelessness, and many others. This isn't to say that every inmate falls into the category of being difficult. For some reason, the most unexpected things happen in prisons and jails.

Constitutionally, inmates should be provided with reasonable medical and mental health care. That means you can't lock them up and throw away the key. Many times, there are dental issues, pending surgeries, medications, serious medical and mental health conditions, and many more circumstances that should be considered and often continued if possible.

Not all medications that a patient takes on the streets will be allowed in a correctional facility. There are hundreds of different prisons and jails throughout the United States. This includes Federal prison/jails, state prisons, and many other forms of detention centers. Each facility will do things a little differently from one to another. This could be based on region, size, beliefs, medical knowledge, medical personnel, administration, financial, and many other things. In essence, what works for one jail may not work for another.

Medicine inside correctional facilities can be exciting, difficult, and even disturbing. It is rare when someone is satisfied with the level of care they are receiving, even if it is exceeding the standards available. Lawsuits are often brought against medical personnel, prisons, and jails. Some of these are for a good reason, but many are not.

The truth of the matter is that inmates are people and should be treated with appropriate medical care regardless of the crimes that brought them to the correctional facilities. On the opposite side of the coin, the medical staff is often attacked, berated, threatened, and more when they are trying to do the best job they can.

The following stories are intended to give the reader a picture into some of the crazier and unbelievable aspects of medicine. These stories are based on true situations, but many things have been changed to protect the patient. Some stories have been combined or changed to give the reader a better understanding and picture of the world of correction medicine.

To our knowledge, all patients involved received excellent health care.

Please enjoy!!

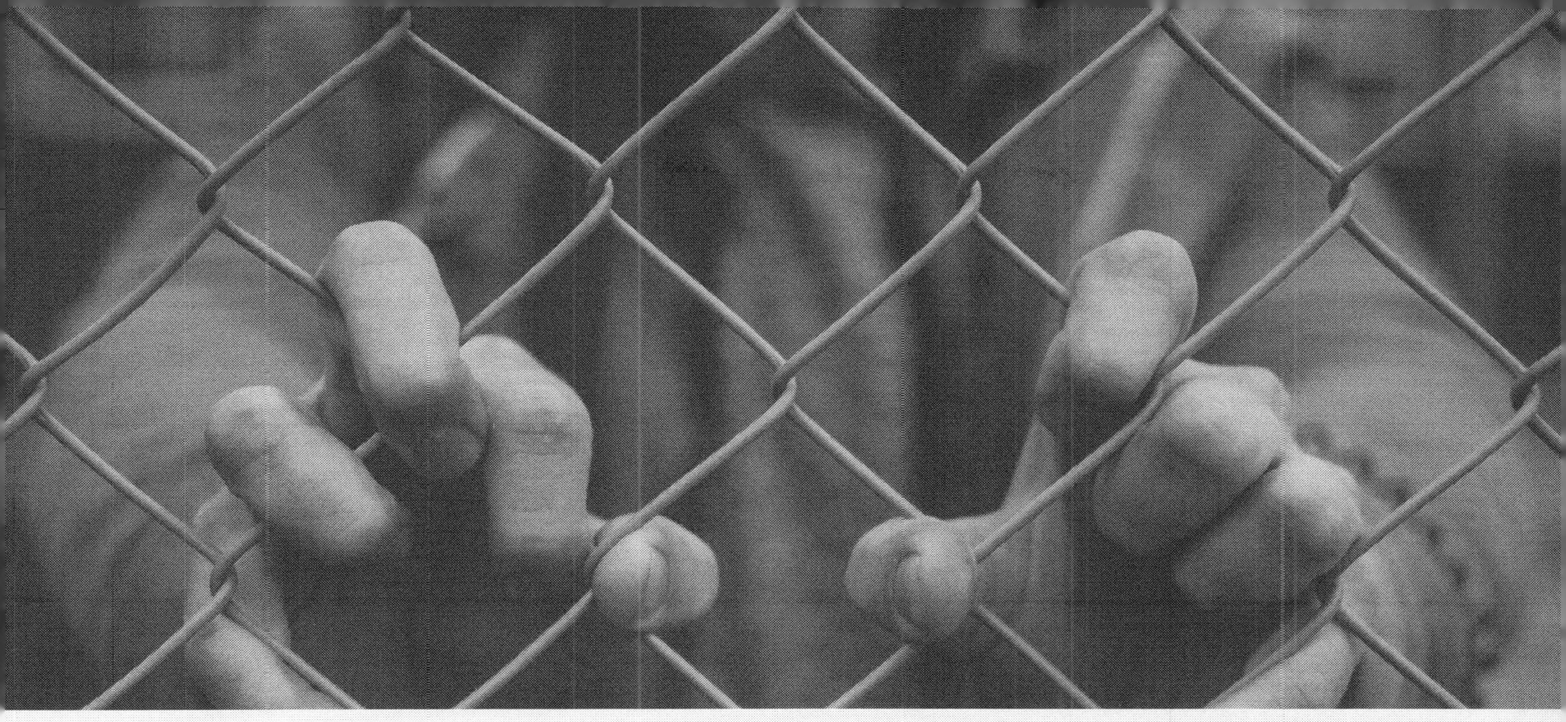

Introduction

This is Volume 3 of Tales of the Exam Room. So far, most of our stories have come from clinics, emergency rooms, and such. Volume 3 is much different. These stories come from Prisons and Jails around the county. These stories are substantially more graphic than the previous stories. Readers beware.

The medical stories that we share are designed to better represent what medical professionals deal with when it comes to patients and their families. They are often trying to make the best decision in a less than favorable circumstance.

These stories are real – but some of the details have been changed or modified. This may or may not include locations, dates, times, names, and some of the specifics. Often, we get asked why we change these things. Obviously, we are trying to protect the patient's identities. Specific things said are often too graphic or to profane to place in this type of a book. Some of the stories have happened more than once. We combine some of the items to allow for a fuller story.

In all of our books, we are trying to help the readers understand the love that medical professionals have for both their patients and the medicine around them. Being part of an unusual case or situation -if handled properly, can be extremely satisfying. That doesn't mean that we "hope" for bad things to happen. The art of medicine is seldom black and white. There are many reasons why it is called "practicing" medicine. Sometimes, decisions are made in a split moment, and what works for one patient may or may not work for another.

Patients are people. They are not always defined by their medical conditions. But some stories touch us in ways that unless you were there, it is hard to understand. Furthermore, not everyone thinks the same. Some people will leave the hospital AMA (Against Medical Advice) and refuse procedures that could save their lives. Other patients will self-sabotage or misunderstand what is being recommended. These stories try to capture the lives and choices of several different individuals.

As mentioned in Volume One and Two - This is a fictional piece and is mainly for entertainment. Our goal is to allow you to see into the world of medicine and some of the bizarre encounters that have happened. We are not trying to poke fun at anyone specifically. If your story happens to line up exactly with ours (Trust me...we are not that good), it's probably more of a coincidence. There are some medical truths and teachings that have been added for the readers' benefit.

Feel free to Join Us for additional medical stories at examroomtales.com

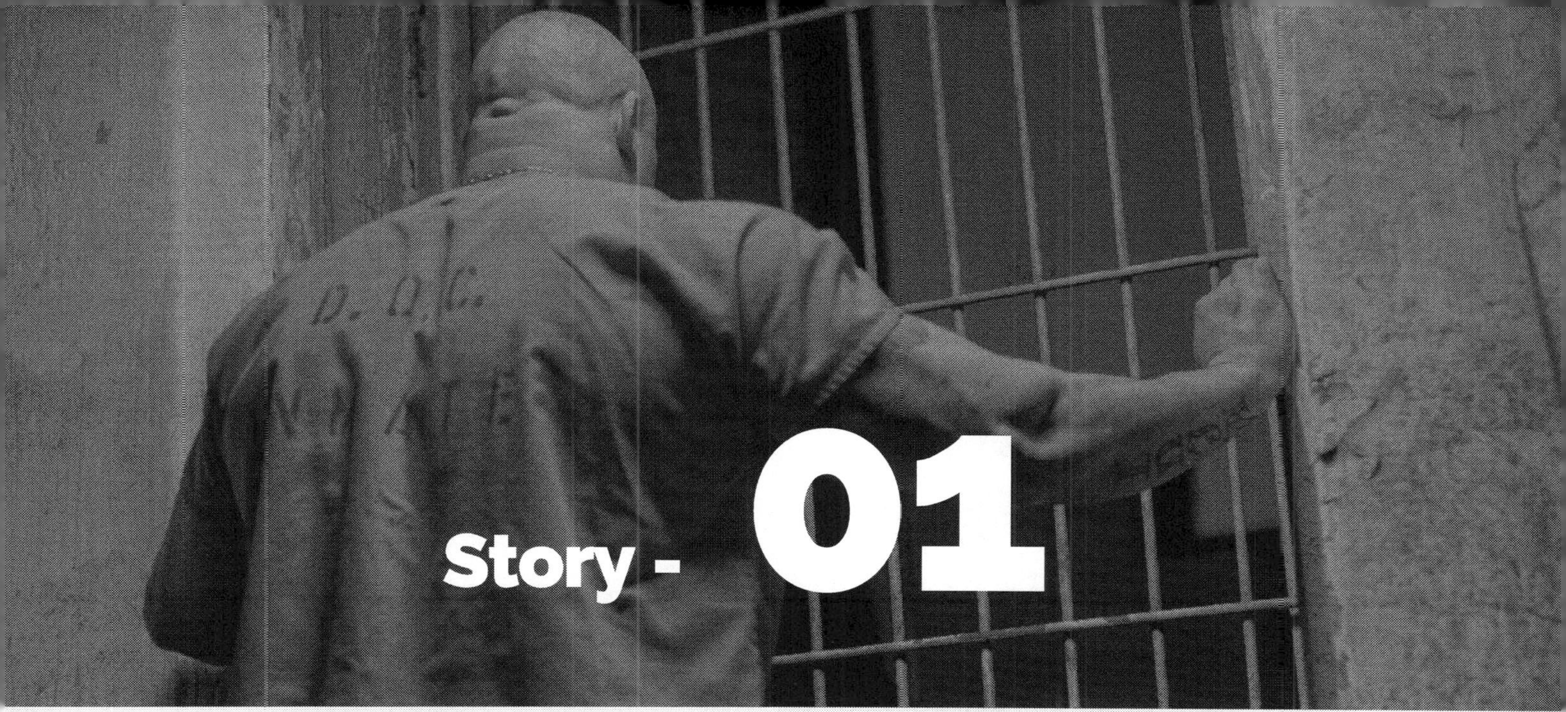

Story - 01

Are There Crazy People in Prison?

The call that came in over the radio was the first significant incident of the day. It was early in the morning; we were just about to finish our shift and were making our last rounds of our shift. The voice was frantic when it said, "We have an emergency. An inmate is standing in a pool of blood. He won't respond, but he is breathing. We need medical, mental health if available, and more officers."

The officers called the medical staff, and several people rushed out of the main medical area and down several halls. They pushed a gurney and a portable three lead EKG machine. They had two or three bags of supplies. On these types of calls, you never know what you are going to find. The medical staff had to pass through three or four different security checkpoints in order to arrive at the cell of the patient in question.

Our prison holds nearly 10,000 inmates, and we have several different sections of the prison and many different buildings. From my understanding, this is pretty common. Men and women are divided as well as some of the more violent criminals. In this particular section of the prison, we mostly have inmates that will serve less than five years. Like most, our facility has a medical staff on-site at all times, which is very helpful. The call came at 4 am. I arrived early for my shift in medical, and along with four nurses, we hurried to the section, unsure what to expect. My colleague pushed the gurney to the side of the cell, out of view. Three officers were already positioned outside the cell door waiting for us.

We quickly learned that the patient was in a cell by himself. He had responded, during the night, to some of the other safety checks. It was an hour or two before breakfast was to be served. When the officer making rounds saw that the inmate was standing, it surprised him. That's when he noticed the blood. Safety in these circumstances is essential. This includes officers, medical staff, and the patient. The officers preach over and over – you never enter a cell by yourself. The medical staff is not allowed into cells, even in medical emergencies, unless the situation is safe. We can't help the patient if we aren't safe. This may mean that things get worse. That may be hard for some people to understand.

In this circumstance, Mr. Fedorov was in a cell by himself. None-the-less, the doors were not opened because the inmate was refusing to cuff up. At this point, he was refusing to answer any question from the officers. He was standing with his back to the cell's door, five feet away from the door. In typical fashion, this section of the prison, the doors had the well-known bars from ceiling to floor. I was leading this call and stepped forward to talk with Mr. Fedorov. He was mumbling to himself, and nothing he said made sense. At his feet, there was a small pool of blood. He was fully dressed in a prison outfit that was one-piece that went over his shoulders and to his feet. It buttoned in the front. I couldn't tell where the bleeding was coming from.

I was the charge nurse and rushed forward. I began asking Mr. Fedorov what was wrong. He refused to answer. Again, and again, I asked him several different questions. It seemed to me that he was in a daze, and I'm not sure how much of what I was asking made sense. Soon the officers were yelling, and Mr. Fedorov flinched. This seemed to get his attention. He didn't turn around, but his head turned as if he was trying to look at me.

I said, "Mr. Fedorov, we are here to help. Will you let us help you?"

Mr. Fedorov said, in a thick and throaty accent, "I think I need some help."

"Can you tell me what is wrong? Why are you bleeding?"

"Because I am strong, and I help people."

"Are you alright? Does anything hurt?"

"I am close to heaven. Can you see me? Am I floating?"

"I see you, Mr. Fedorov. I am here to help."

"That's nice."

"Can you walk back to the cell door and let the officer cuff you?"

"Will you hurt me?"

"Not at all. In fact, we are going to move you to a better living area."

"I want that. Thank you."

Mr. Fedorov slowly began shuffling his feet. I was fearful that he would trip over his clothes or something and fall back into the door. Fortunately, that did not happen. When Mr. Fedorov was cuffed, and the scene was determined to be safe, he was pulled from his room and placed on the gurney. The front buttons of his jumpsuit were buttoned, but a dark stain of blood was apparent. It started in his stomach and continued down both legs. I couldn't see what exactly was taking place. Mr. Fedorov's face was white, but he smiled brightly at me.

"What happened?" I asked.

"I am so strong and powerful,"

"But what about the blood?"

"It's beautiful."

An officer asked, "Can we change his cuffing to let him lay down on the gurney?"

The Sergeant said, "That's fine. Be ready if he does anything."

Mr. Fedorov was compliant with all the commands, and soon we were pushing him back to our central medical area. Our prison started as one large building that enabled medical and other areas to respond quickly. As we have grown, additional add ons have been required. It took several minutes to get him back to our medical area. Other nurses were checking vitals, pulses, temperature, and such. I walked next to Mr. Fedorov - but he refused to say anything more.

Once we arrived in medical, the patient was transferred to a medical bed. Soon, one of the providers came in for an evaluation. I remained in the room to assist with any request by the doctor. Mr. Fedorov refused to say anything at first. The doctor asked several questions, but Mr. Fedorov remained silent. Soon, I started asking the same questions. For some reason, he would only answer what I asked. The doctor nodded at me to continue.

I said, "Mr. Fedorov, you are bleeding. Do you know how that happened?"

"I certainly do. As sure as I know my own daughter."

"Can you tell us?"

"I will tell you. You will be amazed at my strength and courage."

"I bet I will. What exactly happened?"

Mr. Fedorov began telling a story. He said, "It started last night. I had a good meal and a good sleep. I started to feel unsettled in the middle of the night. I woke up a few times. The third time, I prayed that I would be able to go back to sleep, and I received an immediate answer." At this point, Mr. Fedorov lay his head back and screamed, "Love you, brother," at the top of his voice.

The doctor and I exchanged a look.

After a few more minutes, I asked, "How your prayer answered?"

"In fact, it was. But not by whom I thought would answer me. I was visited by my brother-in-law, Igor. The last time I saw him was ten years. In fact, he died just a few years back. It was he who came and visited me."

"Okay. What happened next?"

"Igor asked me a bunch of questions. He wanted to know how I was doing. He was shocked that I was in prison. He told me that I didn't belong there."

"I see. What else?"

"He asked me if I love him." At this moment, Mr. Fedorov glanced up at me, directly into my eyes. His eyes were starting to water. He said, "I told Igor that I loved him more than my Babushka's Borsht." (At the time, I had no idea what he was saying. I later learned that Babushka is like an older woman or grandmother. Borsht is a soup with beets. Sounds very gross to me.)

I asked, "Is that a lot?"

"Lots of love, honey." He winked at me.

I gathered my own courage and asked. "Then what happened?"

"Igor asked me again if I love him, and again I told him that I did. I began pleading with him for me to show him how much I loved him." Mr. Fedorov smiled wistfully and continued, "Prove it, Igor said to me. and I said that I would do anything. He kept saying - Prove it - over and over again."

At this point, I didn't like where this was going. The doctor was trying his best not to laugh, but he nodded in my direction to continue.

Mr. Fedorov said, “Igor told me to remove something that was valuable to me and cast it away. I didn’t know what he meant at first, but the truth eventually came to me.”

“You needed to cast something away?” Against my better judgment, I asked, “What valuable thing did you case away?”

“My most important treasure, my testicle. I used a spork and just about succeeded.”

The doctor performed an exam, and sure enough, his testicle was partway down his pant leg. He had gashed into the skin and caused serious harm and injury. I had never seen anything like this before. It was still attached and bleeding. There was blood everywhere. I started an IV as the doctor worked to put a bandage on the wound. It took some time to get the bleeding slowed. He was quickly sent to the local hospital, and he required surgery to remove the damaged testicle because it had been so injured. The opposite testicle was monitored closely over the next several days but turned out to be fine. He was in prison for several more years, always bragging about what he was willing to do to show love.

The next part is what I add to anyone who ever asks me to hear a prison story. “They ask - Are there crazy people in prison? Yes - there are people who are half nuts.”

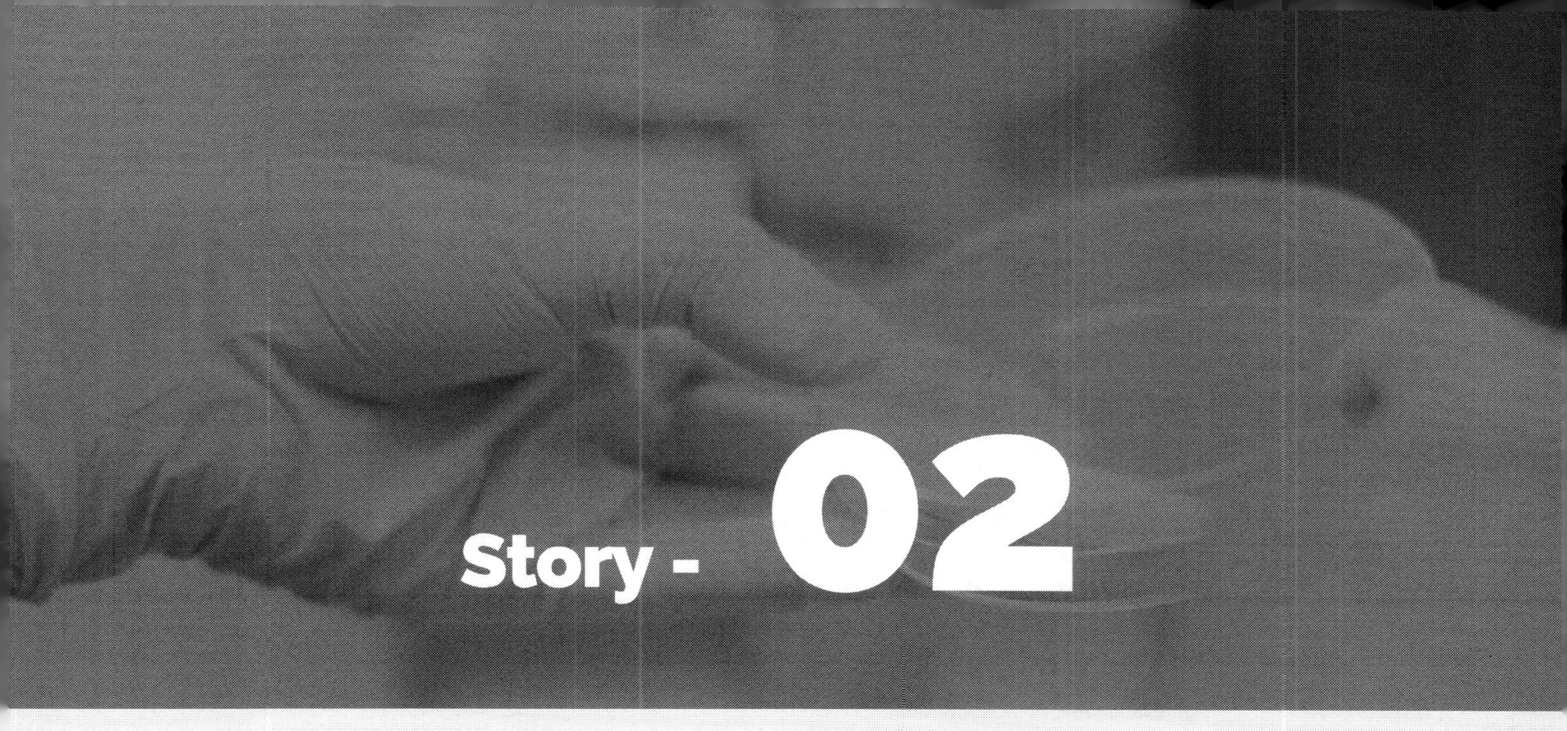

Story - 02

X-ray Shows Hidden Treasure

In most prisons, you have a medical area designated to treat those with the most severe medical conditions. Often, but not always, this area is called the infirmary. There can be a nursing station, several exam rooms, several cells designed to have the sickest of the sick housed in an easily accessible area by the medical staff. In our prison - we have eight exam rooms and over thirty such cells. Some of the housed inmates in this area are so sick that they will never be housed anywhere else in the prison. They often need one-on-one care by a nursing assistant (CNA), medical assistant (MA), or nurse. We have four providers that are assigned to this area. It is often difficult to be assigned to such an area for a prolonged period of time, so we rotate these providers each week.

The medical area also has exam rooms that allow for emergency patients not housed in the infirmary to be seen and scheduled. These types of patients could also include a patient with an infection, a stroke, elevated blood sugars, a laceration that requires sutures, or many other such problems. The medical unit, especially during the day, can be a very busy area. At night, providers are on call to deal with any emergencies. Nurses are on staff to perform assessments and call for orders.

One week, a few years ago, I was assigned as the provider in charge of the "walk-ins," and I was assigned to be on call for that same week. I would see patients during the day and address any issues at night. If something needed to be seen the next morning, they would be added to my scheduled. My colleague was assigned to those housed in the infirmary and in other areas of the prison.

My second day, a patient - Mr. Duncan - came into the medical unit with a complaint of Kidney stones. This is a common complaint either due to the lack of water being consumed or the desire for pain medications. It is important to work them up as you would anywhere else. He had blood in his urine and some flank pain. His vitals were normal. I spent some time with him, trying to see if anything else could be the problem. It was weird, Mr. Duncan came across as if he was holding out on information. He would tell me a little, then wait. It took him over an hour to urinate for the sample that we needed. On the third time, I went into the exam room, he suddenly changed his mind about everything, refused treatment, and wanted to leave the medical area as quickly as possible.

On my third day, I stepped into my next patient's room and was surprised to see Mr. Duncan was back. It was apparent that he wasn't excited that I was the provider seeing him. This time, he was here for a skin burn. He insisted that his kidney problems had resolved, and he assured me that he must've passed the stone. His main concern for today was that he'd dropped some hot water onto his foot. Sure enough, he had a large blister on his foot. It was a second-degree burn, and there was a large blister - larger than a golf ball on the top of his foot. Mr. Duncan expressed a desire to break the blister, but I strongly encouraged him to avoid doing so. I explained that breaking the blister could put the area of skin at risk of an infection. He was advised that he would be given some specific burn cream, and he would be ordered for daily dressing changes. I gave him some pain medications, and he was very appreciative of the care he was given.

On my fourth day, the first name I searched for was Mr. Duncan. Sure enough, he was on my list again–this time for an infection. The area affected had not been specifically outlined in the charting. I entered the exam room, and this time, Mr. Duncan was overtly upset that I was there. He demanded, "I want to see someone else. Isn't there anyone else?"

I replied, "Nope. Just me for today. Where is this infection?"

"On my foot," he said.

"Did you break the blister?" I asked.

"It broke on its own," he said, clearly uncomfortable.

As I evaluated the blister, I was surprised by the amount of redness that was there. The blister had indeed been broken, but it also appeared that there was a large amount of sand and dirt embedded in the wound. It was as if he had taken soil and rubbed it into the wound purposefully. It took nearly an hour to clean out the wound properly. Next, the wound was bandaged, and I ordered Mr. Duncan an antibiotic. I explained the dressing change procedure and the importance of taking his medications entirely.

As he left, he said. "Sorry for the inconvenience. I promise you won't see me tomorrow."

True to his word, Mr. Duncan was not on my list the following day. However, three hours after my shift had ended, and I was at home, I received a phone call from the prison explaining that Mr. Duncan had reported that he had an infection on his skin, caused by a burn that we were refusing to treat. He had been brought up to medical. I was sent a picture. His skin, if possible, appeared worse than it had the day before.

Additionally, he was reporting a long-standing history of kidney stones and that no one at the prison was helping him at all. The nurse had dutifully reviewed the chart and had seen how much we had done for him. The nurse had observed him for an hour and had cleaned his wound, and had his cell searched for the antibiotics. He hadn't taken a single dose. The nurse reported that the odd thing was that Mr. Duncan was trying to negotiate that he could stay in medical until eight pm, and he wouldn't file a complaint against the medical staff. All he wanted to do was to "recover" in the medical unit. Instead, he was admitted to the infirmary until I could see him the next morning. Mr. Duncan was furious that we were making him stay overnight in the infirmary.

Around five in the morning, the same nurse called back, explaining that Mr. Duncan had pushed a button and reported stomach pain, hip pain, and vomiting. The nurse said that Mr. Duncan was actually presenting as someone extremely sick. They pulled him out of his room, and he was having trouble walking and was holding his stomach. I ordered some STAT labs and an abdominal and hip X-ray. I finished getting ready and headed into the prison.

By the time I arrived, Mr. Duncan was crying and screaming that he was in pain. At first, we were again thinking about kidney stones. The X-ray had just been done, and I waited to look at the films. The surprising aspect was that Mr. Duncan had tried to initially refuse the X-ray, but the nurses had been able to convince him to allow it. When I first looked at the film, I was shocked at what I found.

I quickly went to talk with Mr. Duncan. "Tell me what is really going on. I have looked at the X-ray."

Mr. Duncan explained, through gritted teeth, "Totally not a big deal. I knew my cell area was going to get searched this week. I bit my cheek and spit into my urine to make it show that I had blood. I was hoping to meet one of my friends up here in medical. He was going to complain about some chest pain. That didn't work, so I poured hot water onto my foot. It caused a blister, and I knew that the nurse would allow me to come up to medical."

"We're you trying to injure yourself?"

"Yes and no. Check it out - I really needed to see my friend. I was holding onto something for him."

"Go on."

"He didn't show up again. So I got pissed. I was holding it for him in the first place."

"You broke your blister and poured sand into it?" I asked.

"I didn't have a choice. I couldn't be caught with this thing. Also, my friend really needed it. We planned on both coming up after hours last night. I'm not sure what happened to him."

"Are you going to tell me his name?"

"No way. I'll deny that I ever said anything. In fact, I'll say that someone put it up there while I was sleeping here in medical."

Shaking my head, I added, "I'm not here to get anyone in trouble. I just want to help you."

"Then do something!" he shouted.

"Can you remove it on your own?"

"Yesterday I could. Last night though, it wouldn't come out."

"Why hide it in your rectum?"

"That's one of the only places the officers won't check. It took some practice, but it works really well."

"Not a smart idea, especially if you can't get it out."

"I see that now. It's not like I ever planned on it getting stuck. Now my stomach hurts really bad."

I pulled out a copy of the X-ray. "If I am not mistaken, that is a tattoo gun that is stuck in your intestines. It looks like you used a Walkman to make it work."

"This is why I didn't want to get the X-ray," he muttered.

I continued, "Not only is the tattoo gun stuck, but it also looks like you perforated your intestines. Your large intestines."

"What does that mean?"

I put on a glove and pulled too hard. One of my fingers broke through the glove. I said, "A perforation is when there is a tear in your bowel. Essentially, stool is leaking into your abdominal cavity. It is extremely dangerous. That's why you are getting so sick. That's why your stomach hurts so badly and why you've been throwing up."

"How can we fix it?"

"The nurses have already called an ambulance. It looks like you are on the way to the hospital and getting surgery. All to hide a tattoo machine."

"My friend is that good at tattoos," Mr. Duncan said as if his own life meant nothing. "What will happen to the tattoo gun?"

"The hospital will likely keep it."

"I refuse to go. I am sure I can get it out on my own. Just give me some lube or something."

"Then, you will likely die."

Grumbling, he said, "This is the stupidest thing ever. It's like you are punishing me."

Mr. Duncan required two surgeries to remove the machine and repair the intestine. He developed another infection post-operatively, and this resulted in a third surgery. It took him approximately six months to fully recover.

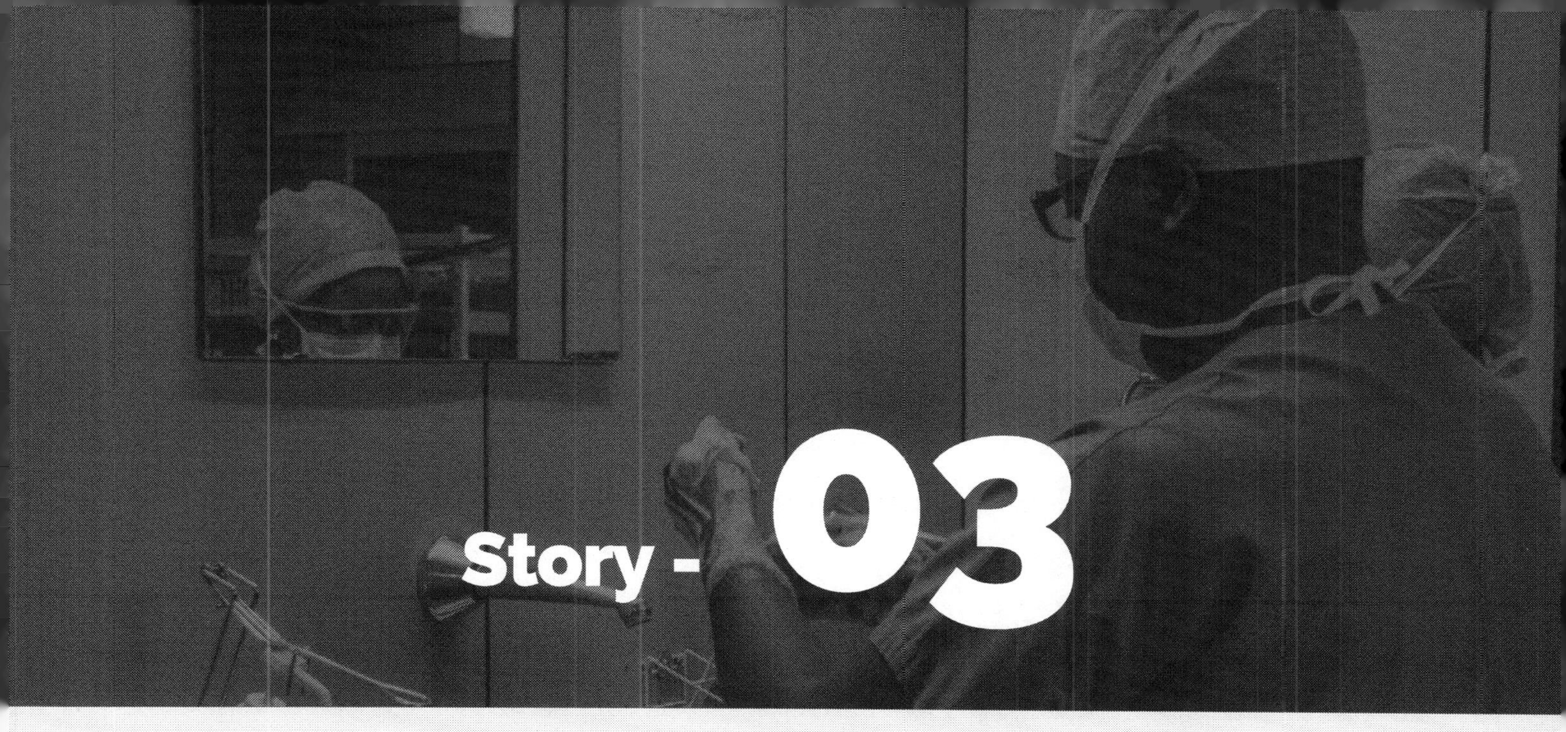

Escape If you Can, My Candy Princess!!

There are several things that I loved and hated about being a student studying medicine. There was so much information that I was in survival mode most of the time. I had a lot of great teachers and experiences. One of the experiences I'll never forget is when, as a student, I was asked to visit a large prison for three days. The prison was the last place that I wanted to do some of my clinical experience. I hated the idea of being locked down in a concrete building with people who had done terrible things.

On my first day, I was waiting in my car, in a line to get into the entrance of the prison. I had to wait for over an hour as all the cars were being searched. An officer with drug dogs began circling around all the cars in front of me. I had no clue what was going on. Eventually, they came to my car and explained that they were looking for drugs being smuggled into the prison. I wanted to turn the car around right then and there and go home. That was a lot to handle. Trust me, it only got worse from there.

When they closed the door to the outside world, and I was locked up with a bunch of criminals, I thought I was going to have a panic attack. I met some of the strangest and scary people inside prison. But I also met the most normal-appearing individuals with problems that were so routine that they could be you or me. In fact, most of those that I met were kind and respectful. The ones that weren't were really off the wall. At the end of my experience, I learned so much about the prison and the crazy medical things that happen that I appreciate those that work there full time. That line of work is just not for me.

My story is about a patient that I saw on my third and last day. By that point, I had met and talked with over a hundred inmates. I learned their backstories and was surprised to see all the damage in their lives that led to them being locked up. On my last day, I was allowed to go in alone and ask the patient several questions.

As I walked into the room, the patient had shackles around his waist and was chained to the wall. He couldn't move more than a few inches. He had his arms clear, and he could move them a few inches, but I was safe. I was able to have plenty of space to use the computer, review his history, medications, and such. Surprisingly, after three days, I felt less afraid in these exam rooms than almost anywhere else in prison. I was tasked to see if I could see any mental health or medical problems and evaluate his medications.

The male, around twenty-five, was muscular, short, and in good shape. He was smiling and was kind when I asked him questions. He had some facial tattoos as well as tattoos on his arms. I guessed that he was likely a part of a gang. He had a rough exterior, but he smiled and said hi. Inside the prison, some individuals, especially, but not always the men, whistle or say crude remarks. I was hoping that this visit would be better than some of the others I had experienced. For the first few minutes, this patient was the kindest I had seen so far at the prison. He would say, "Yes ma'am," or "No ma'am," to everything. He seemed to contemplate every question I asked. We will call him Jose.

After the basic history and medication questions, I had started asking him about any treatment history, either commitments or otherwise. He answered these questions extensively. He had been institutionalized three separate times. He was so clear in his thoughts and his honesty that I was surprised. He didn't appear confused or delusional.

However, not long after, I noticed something change in his facial features. Even to this day, I'm not sure what it was. He asked, "Do you know what time it is?"

"About four-thirty."

"Oh, splendid. Dinner will be served soon. I love the food here."

"Really?" I asked. "I've never heard that before."

"Oh yes. It makes you big and strong. Nobody will mess with you if you are big and strong. The food here isn't as good as one of my candies."

"I guess." I sat back in my chair and tried to understand the change I was seeing. I pulled up his chart again and reviewed his medical medications. I said, "Having you been taking your meds?"

"Of course," Jose said. "They are also the candies of my life."

I was suddenly interested in where this conversation would go. He was pleasant enough, but I was just starting to sense that there was something off about him.

Jose added, "Can you allow me to have a bag full of candies tonight?"

I said, "If you remember, I am a student. I can ask your question to my trainer. She will come in and ask you some more questions if she needs to. Is that okay?"

"Without a doubt," Jose said. "You are almost as pretty as one of my candies."

"Thank you," I said hurriedly. I had asked this question before, but I asked it again, "Are you having any mental health or medical issues?"

"Not. At. All. I am in the twilight of my life. I am the moon to your sky. I am the ocean to your land. I am everything, and you complete me."

Now things are starting to get interesting, I thought to myself. Normally, I would've run from the room. He was eying me like candy. I remembered back to my trainer, telling me that this type of thing happens a lot in prison. I was told to stay my ground and push forward. I said, "Your mental health request says that you think that someone is after you."

"Are you a mind reader? I love that gift. I could see it in your color aura when you came into the room. You are right, as always. Someone is after me." Jose leaned forward and winked.

I wasn't sure how much to play into this. His chart reported paranoia, but I had never really seen it before. I was also awestruck at how different he was from just a few minutes ago. I wondered if the sincerity he showed when I first walked in could be faked. I wasn't sure. I decided to continue forward. "Do you know who it is, or does the person stay in the shadows?"

"On Thursdays, he comes out of the shadow, and he has a spider for a head. Usually, he stays in the shadows. He yells at me when I sleep. That's why I need to eat more dinner. If I am big and strong, he won't come after me in the dark. Can I have a candy?"

"Good thing it is Friday," I said. "Do you love or hate spiders?"

"I love them. I would marry them if I could."

"Why does the shadow man frighten you so much?"

"He has traveled through time for centuries to find me. I have a special ability. He wants to take it from me. Do you want to know my special ability?"

I was starting to doubt that I could help Jose. I didn't really know what to do. He now sounded paranoid and mentally unstable. I wasn't sure if I should remain in the same room with him. I didn't think that playing into his delusion would be helpful. Instead, I said, "Abilities should remain hidden, I think. Thanks for talking with me. I probably should be going now." I stood to leave the room.

Suddenly Jose kicked out his feet to prevent me from leaving the exam room. He said, "If you leave before I show you my abilities, the shadow man is going to come after you. I am the only one who knows how to escape him."

Hesitantly, I said, "You do."

In a whisper, he said, "It works every time. But don't tell anyone else."

"If I let you tell me, will you let me leave the room."

"Of course. I just want my princess to be safe. I can teach you the words so that shadow man won't come after you."

Feeling bold, I said, "I know another way for you to escape. I'm sure that if you take your meds, you can. Will you promise to take your meds every day?"

"I promise."

"Okay. What words do I need to say?"

Jose began chanting over and over again. His words weren't making any sense. I noticed that his legs were back in their normal place. I inched forward. Jose's eyes were closed. I was about to escape out of the room when his eyes flung open. And he said loudly, "To escape the Shadow man, you must do as follows!"

Jose lifted his right hand directly in front of his face. The outer portion (not the palm) was facing towards me. He lifted his left hand, and using it, he grabbed the middle finger of his right hand. He shouted, "Escape my candy princess."

To my horror, Jose snapped the middle finger of his hand and broke the finger at one of the joints. He didn't scream out, and his face didn't change. I sprinted from the room and went searching for my trainer. By the time we had returned, with an officer, to his room, Jose had broken two more fingers. They were all pointed sideways. A provider was notified, and Jose was given some medications that calmed him down. The provider spoke with Jose as if he knew him well. Within a few minutes, the patient was sedated, and the doctor had reset each finger. I gaped at the entire interaction.

As the doctor left Jose's room, he said, "Don't worry. This has happened before but not for the last six months. Three finger fractures are more than usual. He must've really liked you."

I was able to see the X-ray of both hands and several that had been done in the past. The patient had three current fractures that were in the healing process and the three new fractures.

The doctor also told me, "This is what he does around this time of the year. It is sort of an anniversary of some sort. His mental health goes down significantly. We try to help him, but he refuses his meds and quickly goes downhill. In a few weeks, he'll be much better and would have never done this. However, this time next year, he might be back to repeating this behavior all over again."

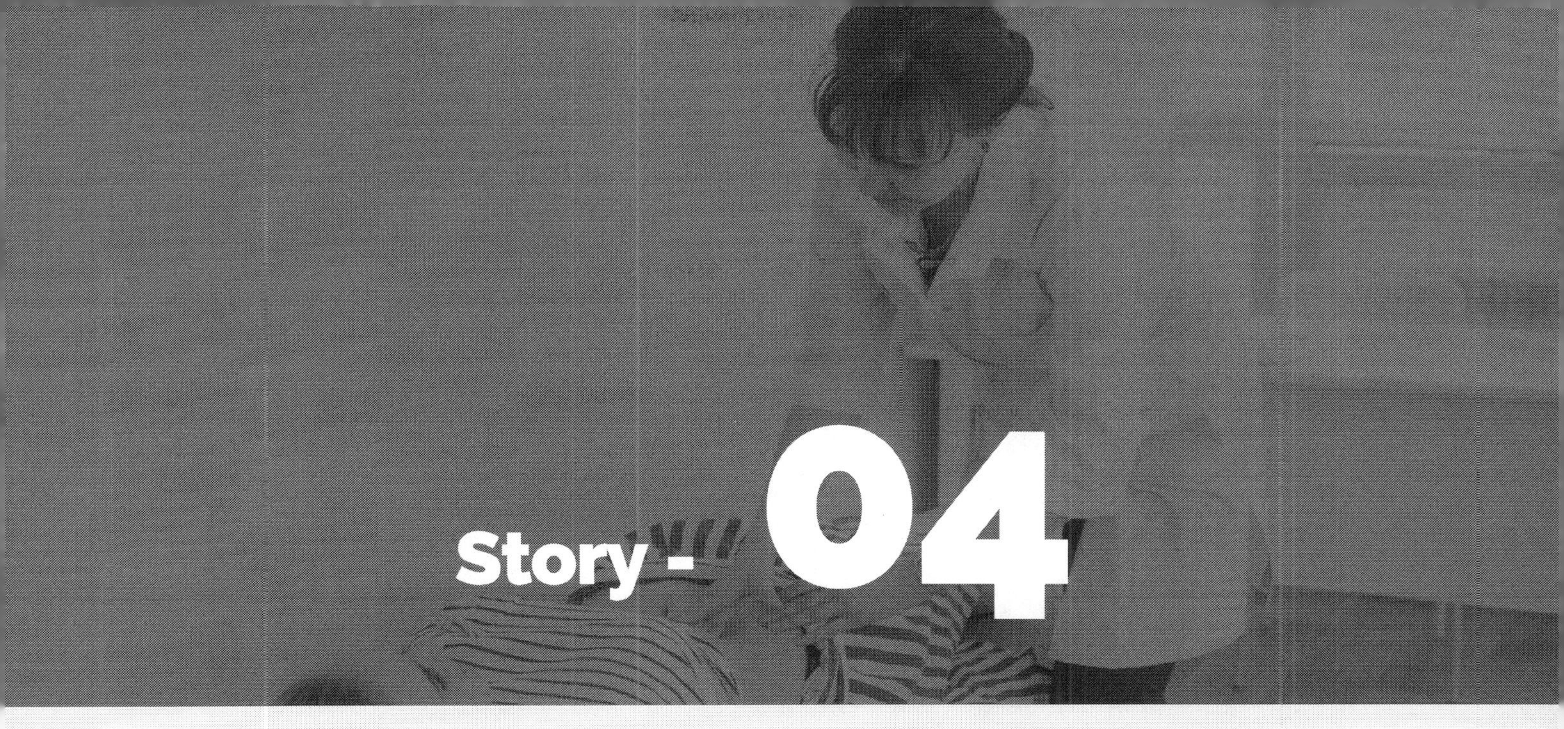

My Stomach Hurts. It's an Emergency.

When you think of a jail, you might be picturing a small building with less than ten cells. Or you might be thinking of something with thousands of inmates such as New York or California. Truthfully, jails across the nation come in varying sizes, shapes, and locations. Some are directly in the city, while others are in small towns or in the middle of nowhere.

Our jail is medium-sized in a town that is also medium-sized but somewhat isolated. We have a small hospital that can treat most issues. A trauma hospital is only a few hours away. Our nurse (myself) goes to the jail three times a week unless there is an emergency. I try to do as much as I can to answer any medical issues, order supplies, and hundreds of other things. If the complaint or situation is more than I can (or should) handle, the medical provider from the local community is called to address the situation. They have their own practice in town, and they come over to the jail whenever needed. Some weeks that is every day while other weeks it could be once a week.

We have a small medical room. Often, I spend some of my time with the officers or other staff, and if there is a question by an inmate, it often goes to the officer first, then to myself. But the inmates have plenty of time during med pass or at other times to ask me questions. Often, the medical staff isn't aware of a problem, especially emergencies, until the officers tell us. In the control room, they open the doors to the jail and monitor areas of the jail. Through cameras, the officers can watch a large amount of the jail. But the cameras can't see everything, and often the officers are walking up and down the halls and performing security checks throughout the facility. Officers have a bunch of overall responsibilities.

One night, I was answering some questions in the control room, and there were a few officers in there with me when one of the inmates started hitting the button in his cell frantically. This button allows the inmate to communicate with the staff. Inmates often hit their buttons for a variety of different reasons. Sometimes they need a shower, or to make a phone call, or to get a book. There are hundreds of buttons pushed every day. Sometimes emergencies do arise. You have to be very careful to manage the buttons. The inmates certainly could spend the entire day pushing the button and reporting some random thing. But they also could be having an emergency and need to be checked on immediately.

When the officer answered, Mr. Alexander, demanded to go to the hospital. The problem was that this was a common occurrence for this patient. In fact, he had been pushing the button so much, he was told that he would get written up if he continued.

This time the officer asked, "What is your reason for needing to go to the hospital?"

"I am a healer," Mr. Alexander exclaimed. "There are sick people at the hospital, and they need my help."

"Are you having a medical emergency?"

"Not yet."

"Let me talk with the nurse, and I'll let you know."

"I am like Jesus, and it's my duty."

"I'll pass it along."

The officer controlling the buttons asked for my opinion. It was clear that we couldn't take him to the hospital, nor should we. Bringing an inmate to the hospital to walk around was out of the question, and Mr. Alexander wasn't experiencing any life-threatening problems himself. He seemed like he wanted a ride out of jail.

The officer answered back, "Sorry. We are unable to take you to the hospital at this time."

"Fine. Have a good night," Mr. Alexander screamed back.

We spent the next twenty minutes giving report and going over several other patients. It was the end of my shift, and there were a few more things I needed to pass along. This is often the process where the officers can ask questions about specific patients, or they can ask about other issues that they might have.

I was getting up to leave when Mr. Alexander hit the button again. I wanted to run from the building before he asked me to come see him again at his cell.

Mr. Alexander said in a shaky voice, "You guys need to come to my cell. There's something wrong, and I need to show you." This time, his accent was thick, and it was hard to understand exactly what he said.

Officer Jenkins, the new officer on shift, asked, "Alexander. Are you having a specific problem? If not, we will be stopping by when we do our rounds."

"Nope. That won't work. You've got to come now."

Officer Jenkins responded, "Are you having an emergency?"

"I am just about to have a big emergency. I want to see the nurse and the Lieutenant now. If you guys don't come down here soon, I am going to hurt myself. You'll have an emergency then, methinks."

Threats of self-harm are often stated in corrections. Sometimes they are said because the individual is angry, and sometimes, they are telling the truth. A patient may report they are having an emergency, but they really want to shower or to get more food. Sometimes they just need someone to talk with or listen to all of their problems. But, as indicated before, sometimes they really have a medical emergency, and they need help now. Me and two officers headed in the direction of Mr. Alexander's cell to make sure everything was alright.

The officer in control monitored the situation as Officer Barrett, the Lieutenant, and I walked to Alexander's cell.

From the control room, over the radio, Officer Jenkins said, "The room is much darker than usual."

Lieutenant Decker asked, "Can you rewind the video to see if something happened?"

As we turned down the corridor of the cells where Mr. Alexander was housed, officer Jenkins said, "The picture isn't really clear, but I think he broke out the lights to his room."

The Lieutenant grumbled, "Just what we need now." Into the radio, she said, "Call Davenport and to meet us at the cell. We could have a situation on our hands."

We weren't sure exactly what was going on, if the inmate would be injured, or something unexpected was going on. At a minimum, Alexander was going to have to cuff up and be removed from his cell in order for staff to search it and make sure it is safe.

Alexander was currently on observation for some behavior issues and was in a cell by himself. This meant he was in a cell with a plexiglass window. This allowed the staff to get a good visual every time they walked past the cell. The camera inside the cell was in a protective case and hard, but not impossible to break. Alexander had been in jail for a few months, and most of the time, he was refusing his medications.

The Lieutenant and Officer Barrett kept off to one side until Officer Davenport arrived. We decided that the plan was for me to talk with Alexander - determine if he was in any danger either from himself or anything that might be broken inside the cell. The officers would remain behind me in case anything happened. If there were no problems, they would determine what their next step was going to be.

I stepped forward but couldn't see Mr. Alexander. The room was pretty dark, and it became apparent quickly that Alexander hadn't broken any lights in the cell. Instead, he had placed wet paper and towels on the light. This caused the room to look darker. I searched the cell and found him standing, huddled against the back wall, naked except his underwear.

"Mr. Alexander, It's Nurse Lucy. Are you alright?"

At the sound of my voice, I could see that Mr. Alexander was sticking his hand into his underwear. I kept calling to him. After a few minutes, he looked over at me and grinned a smile that went from ear to ear.

Mr. Alexander said, "Lucy. So good to see you. I was hoping that you would come and see me Actually, I was praying that you would. The lord answers all my prayers."

"Are you alright? Are you having a medical emergency?"

"Oh, yes. I am alright. But I think that something is wrong with the jail. I just had blood dripping out of my faucet when I was trying to get a drink."

"That sounds bad. I bet we can fix that. I just need you to come over to the window so that I can make sure that you are okay."

Mr. Alexander suddenly slammed his head into the wall two times.

I yelled for him to stop, and he did. I added, "Come over here and let me see how you are doing."

"Okay," he said playfully.

He turned and took two steps towards the window.

"That's good. Keep on coming."

Mr. Alexander stopped near the center of the room. I couldn't see him clearly. But, I didn't see any blood on his forehead or anywhere else. He was walking without any problems. It was clear that he was struggling with his mental health. I asked, "Did you take your meds tonight?"

"Oh. I made them into a stew and snorted them."

"That would be gross. But did you take them?"

"Maybe. What do you think?"

Changing the subject, I said, "Does anything hurt?"

"Oh, my stomach. Dinner was beyond horrible. I think they are trying to torture me, and now I've been having diarrhea all night."

"We can give you something for that. Just come to the door and cuff up, and we can make sure you are alright."

"I am so hungry. It feels like my stomach is withering away."

"What was for dinner?"

Ignoring the question, Mr. Alexander said, "Oh no. More diarrhea." Both of his hands went behind him into his underwear. He bent over, and a loud farting sound burst from Mr. Alexander.

Trying not to laugh, I said, "Do you need to use the toilet?"

Mr. Alexander 's shoulders sank. "Too late." He added, "Now I need a shower. Can you help me?"

"Come over to the door and cuff up."

Standing back up, he pleaded, "So hungry. Please give me some food."

At this point, Mr. Alexander removed both hands from his underwear, and to my horror, they were both filled with a liquidy brown substance. I inadvertently took a step back.

Mr. Alexander began moaning, "Soooo hungry." Taking both hands, full of this brown substance, he began shoving the brown substance into his mouth. One hand full after another. It was dripping off his chin.

I wanted to look away, but I couldn't. It was the worst thing that I had ever seen.

He reached back and took another handful. This time, instead of getting it into his mouth, it hit the side of his face.

I could hear the officers behind me. Officer Barrett had only been at the jail for a week. He was dry-heaving on the floor.

The Lieutenant stepped forward and barked, "Mr. Alexander. This is not the time or place for you to be acting like this. I need you to go wash your hands and cuff up. I am giving you a direct order. You need to comply. We need to clean this cell, and you need to be checked out. This behavior is unacceptable. Stop eating your poo."

And just like that, Mr. Alexander complied. He turned, having brown stained underwear, and walked to his sink. He washed his hands and face and took a long sip of water. As he walked back towards the front of the cell, both hands were placed on his stomach. He kept groaning, "So, hungry."

"Keep coming," demanded the Lieutenant.

Mr. Alexander continued walking. As he reached the front window, the Lieutenant said, "You are going to need to cuff up. Do you understand?"

"Of course, no problem."

I whispered, "Are you going to place your cuffs on his hands?"

"The cuffs can always be washed."

"Gross."

Mr. Alexander began taping the window. He asked, "Can I ask the nurse a question?"

The Lieutenant glanced at me. I said, "I guess." I stepped two very small steps closer.

Mr. Alexander said, "Are there any oatmeal cream pies left on commissary?"

"What are you talking about?" I asked.

He pulled back the covers of his bed and revealed four of five empty plastic wrappers of oatmeal cream pies. He said, "I totally fooled you guys." He took out another cream pie and unwrapped it. He ran to the faucet and poured water over the cream pie, and smashed it together. He returned to the front of the cell and pretended to eat it. He laughed harder than I've ever seen someone laugh. He added, "Did you think that I would really eat my own poop? I'm crazy, but not that crazy." He took his chair and moved it to the center of the room. He stood on it and reaching up, he pulled off the wet towels, and the light in the cell improved dramatically.

As he stepped off his chair, he said, pointing at the ceiling, "That plastic was broken long before I got here."

The Lieutenant was furious. "Are you telling me that this entire thing was a joke?"

"And a darn good one. You should've seen your faces. Especially Nurse Lucy. I thought you were going to have a heart attack."

I still had my hand over my mouth in shock. My mouth was wide open. At first, I wasn't sure if I believed him.

He finished by saying, "I really do need a shower now. But this is the best jail prank ever, and no, I don't need to go to the hospital to heal people."

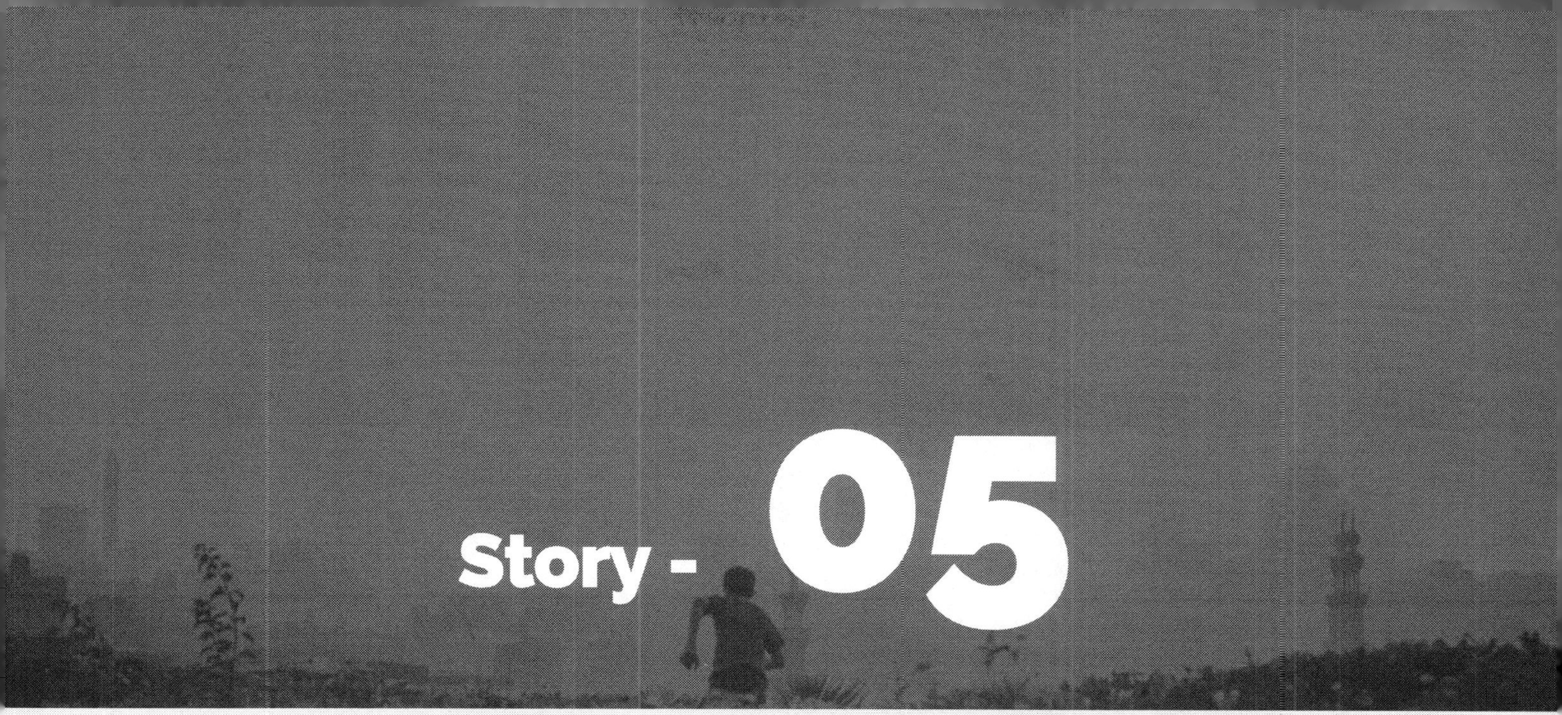

Story - 05

Far From A Leap of Joy

Sometimes in prison, a bad day is made worse by the choices the inmate makes. And really, the occurrence of poor decisions could be applied to any one of us but often inmates' bad choices have severe consequences and longer prison sentences. Sometimes an inmate will get bad news or even good news, and it is as if all common sense flies out the window. This is precisely the case of our most recent story. This story comes to us from a prison with 5,000 inmates on a large campus. There is the main building near the front and center of the area. Behind the building are several smaller and different buildings. These smaller buildings house some of the inmates. This prison isn't on the coast but just a few hours away.

Rico Rodrigues was relaxing and enjoying some time with his friends. It was Friday, and he had spent another week working hard to improve his situation. He had just finished his GED class for the day, as he was working hard to get his high school diploma. It had been a productive day, and he was two weeks away from taking his test. He was satisfied with his effort and felt that he was far ahead of where he needed to be. To be honest, the primary reason he was trying to get his GED was to be able to leave prison early.

He'd been promised by his lawyer that the judge and parole board would look favorably upon him for going to his education classes, working, and taking some religious classes. An extra benefit was that he really wanted to get his high school diploma, and he had plans to use it when he was released. Convicts have a tough time finding jobs after they are released from prison. However, some newer changes give grants and opportunities to convicts, and having a GED would be beneficial.

After class, he was eating and playing cards with his friends, waiting for lunch to be served. In the afternoon, they planned on watching television and more card games. Two back-to-back phone calls changed everything for Rico. The first call was from his lawyer. The judge had reviewed the paperwork submitted to the court last month, and the judge had decided not to give him any additional time off his sentence by getting his GED. It had been about a 50/50 possibility, his lawyer had explained, and Rico was optimistic that he would be given the time cut. It was a hard pill to swallow, and Rico was dazed at this news. Instead of returning to playing cards, he went into his cell to think. If this had been his only phone call, he probably would've escaped without too many problems. Not five minutes later, another inmate came to find him. He was told that he had another phone call.

This time, the call was from his wife. She was waiting for him and was the rock in his life. She wrote to him every week and put money on his books so that he could buy commissary. She sent him books and magazines. She attended all his court meetings. They had talked several times the first six months that he was locked up. They had plans. Three weeks ago, they started planning on where they would live once he was released. She had lined up a few job interviews using the new opportunities that he was given. Best case scenario - he would've been out in three or four months. Now that the judge had eliminated that possibility, he would be out in twelve months. He did not want to give his wife the bad news. He was silent for the first few minutes of the conversation. She must've picked up on something as she was unusually quiet.

Rico asked, "Babe. Is everything alright?"

She answered, "I can't do this anymore."

The line went silent. Rico kept asking what was going on. Finally, his wife's father picked up the phone. Rico was told that his wife was leaving the country with his two sons. Rico wouldn't be told where his wife was going, and no one would be there for him when he was released. Rico had made some huge mistakes, but this news was beyond anything he expected. He argued and yelled and pleaded with the father of his wife. The man pointed out that Rico and his daughter had been married in a backyard near the beach, not two hours away from the Prison that Rico was currently serving. They had never gotten a marriage license or anything else. Rico was told he had no rights to his children or to his wife. He was told he was a criminal and would always be a criminal. As Rico began pleading to talk with his wife again, the man hung up without another word.

Rico was devastated and went into a fog. He became so anxious and upset that he kept thinking that he had to leave and find his wife and convince her to stay. Even days later, he still couldn't remember what happened after the phone call. It was as if his mind shut off.

What really happened after the phone call was caught on several cameras. Rico returned to his cell for lunch and remained there into the early afternoon. He didn't eat or return to playing any cards. Around 3 pm, he and his entire section, were taken to the rec yard for some fresh air and exercise. They had a big field, two basketball courts, a few walls to bounce a small ball against, and other things. Rico spent nearly twenty minutes just walking around the field in a circle. He didn't appear talk to anyone, and when he was approached, he made excuses on why he wanted to be alone.

As a small fight breaks out on the basketball court, Rico is seen leaving the field and starts walking away from all the buildings. A lot is going on, and no one really pays Rico any attention.

He is on the far backside of the prison campus and reaches the back end of the field and walks directly up to the twelve or fifteen-foot fence. Without stopping or taking a second glance, he starts climbing up the fence. He climbs easily and without any problems. He makes it near the top of the fence, about a foot away. On top of the fence, there is a fair amount of razor wire that is rolled over itself the length of the fence. Somehow,

Rico slithers and crawls up the remainder of the fence and through the wire. From the camera angle, it is hard to tell how much he is cut. There is more razor wire on the other side of the fence. Instead of climbing through this wire, he jumps over it and falls down towards the ground on the other side of the fence. He lands feet first and doesn't fall or even stumble.

He is now in "no man's land." This area is the ten feet of ground between the inner fence and the outer fence. Even weeks later, Rico can't tell me how he feels, because he doesn't remember doing this. Back to the camera, there are no alarms sounding for a full five minutes. But Rico is unable to take another step, and he just stands there. It doesn't take long for several officers to arrive on the scene. Guns are drawn, and a gate is opened, and officers rush in, and Rico is immediately cuffed. There are shouts and commands, but Rico doesn't move the entire time. A medical van is called to help Rico, but he refuses and finally begins walking back towards the main building, where the medical area is located. It is a full ten-minute walk back to an area, and Rico is escorted immediately to medical.

An officer told me that as they walked, Rico kept saying, "Just take me back to my cell."

When Rico arrives in the medical department, an entire team is ready for him. At the door of the main building, Rico is placed onto a gurney. By the time he enters medical, he is screaming and yelling. He isn't upset that he can't walk, but rather, the pain has started to overwhelm him. The adrenaline of the situation has finally worn off, replaced by pain that is beyond our understanding. Two nurses and I quickly attend to Rico. Pain medications and IV placement are the first things given. Pulling up Rico's pant legs - it is evident that both legs have buckled considerably. A jump from that distance would injure anyone. But looking at Rico's legs, I knew that he had broken both of them and that he needed treatment far beyond the scope of the prison. We did the best that we could to get Rico settled, and an ambulance was called. The surprising thing was that he only had a few cuts on his arms, neck, and top of the head. At the time, I didn't even know that it was from a fence.

Once Rico left on the ambulance, one of the Captains came into medical and said that the security video had been reviewed. We didn't completely know what had happened as we were treating Rico. We had been told that he had likely jumped from somewhere. When the story was told, everyone was in complete shock at what had happened. Many of the staff knew Rico pretty well and were surprised that he acted in this way. Others wondered how close Rico must have come from getting shot. He had been found trying to escape the prison. They don't take escape attempts lightly. No one had ever climbed over the fence before. Others had tried going up the one side, but no one had ever managed to get to the other side. But by far, the most surprising thing was that Rico had landed, walked to medical, having shattered both of his legs. He had probably lost a half-inch of his height due to this injury.

A short time later, Rico arrived at the hospital in shackles and with several officers. After his initial exam, it wasn't long before he was taken to the OR (operating room) for emergency surgery. He spent several days in the hospital and required a few different surgeries. He needed significant treatment and rehab to be able to walk again. It took over six months for things to even start to improve. The information came back even worse when he was given an extra five years - for a charge of trying to escape. All-in-all, it was one of the most remarkable stories that I've ever seen.

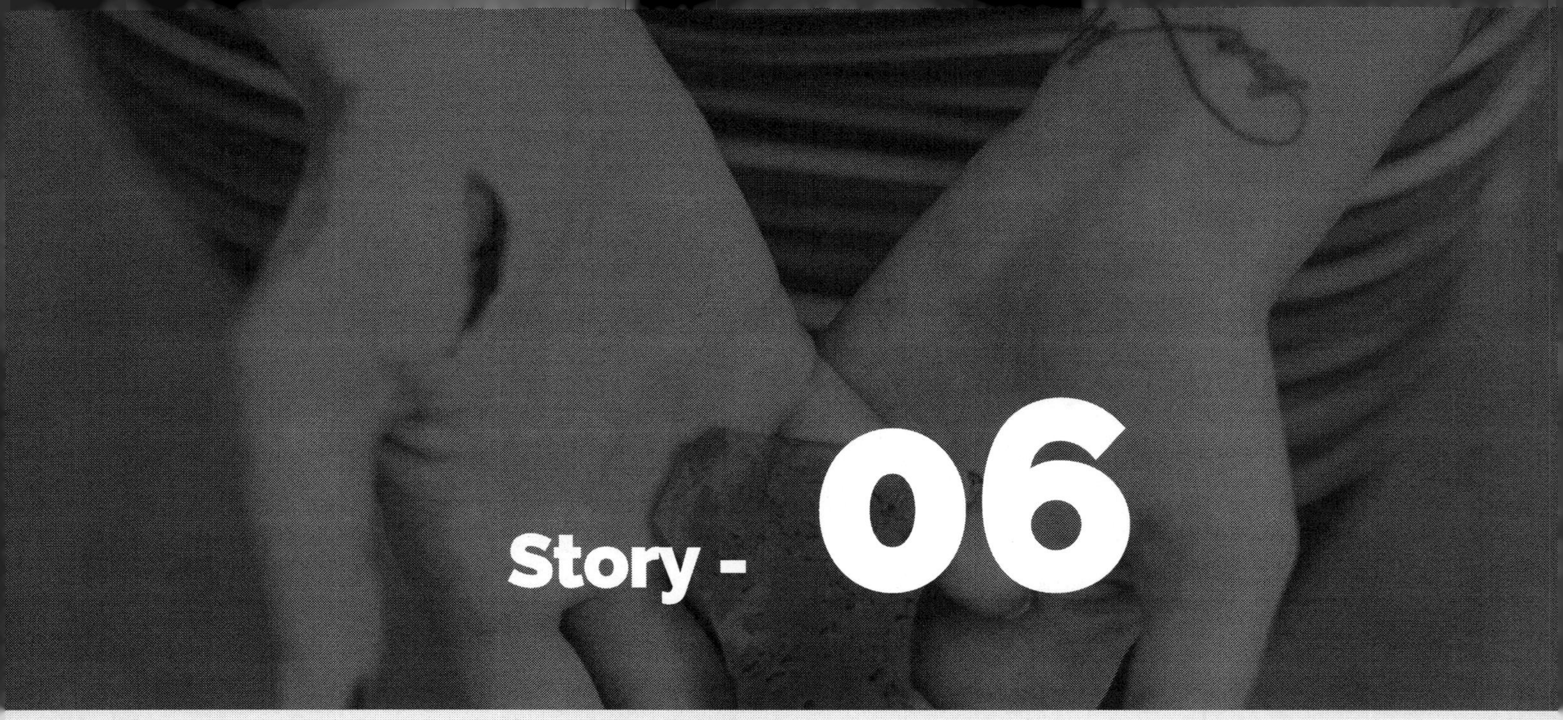

She Cut Her Finger On a Can; It's no Big Deal

Feeding inmates in a large prison facility can be a very difficult thing to do. Often we don't have enough staff to cover all the shifts and prepare all the food. When you have thousands of inmates and several different kitchens, we learned long ago, that the only option was to have inmates become kitchen workers. This brings a large amount of both good and bad to the situation. Some days you aren't sure how the entire prison doesn't burn down.

Teaching inmates how to cook has a lot of benefits such as, learning to work with others, and especially the importance of avoiding the boredom that comes with being in prison. Often, they can eat food that they normally wouldn't be served. But, there can be a lot of consequences as well. There are a fair number of inmates that get into fights in the kitchen. They often talk a lot and sometimes their mouths (or something else) can get them in trouble. Add in missing items, smuggling of things, workplace injuries, and a whole lot more that you don't want to even think about.

Our prison has both men and women. They aren't in the same area or the same building, in fact, they are on opposite sides of the entire prison. We have eight kitchens for the men and two for the women.

As a nurse, I was in the medical room, helping with a dressing changes when I received a phone call from an officer in the female kitchen.

The male officer said, "Hey, this is officer Reynolds, and we need someone to come out to the hallway leading to the kitchen. One of the girls cut the tip of her finger on a can."

"An aluminon can," I replied. "How much bleeding is there? How does it look?"

Officer Reynolds replied, "I actually haven't seen the injury. I am just relaying what my partner said."

"Okay. I'll grab some supplies and head on over."

It took five minutes to gather everything I needed and another five minutes to walk through the open courtyard to the kitchen. Ten feet away from the doors leading to the kitchen, two girls came running out of the building. They refused to look at me. My first thought was that they were going to be late getting back to their cells before the lockdown for dinner began. If they were late, they could lose some privileges.

As I entered the building, I heard ear-piercing cries coming from the hallway ahead. I hurried forward to find where they were coming from. There was no one in the hall where officer Reynolds had indicated the inmate would be waiting. I could see a few drops of blood on the floor. I searched frantically for a few minutes. The screams would come and go. Finally, I tracked down a group of girls inside one of the bathrooms.

Inside the bathroom, there was more blood on the floor. Three girls were at the sink frantically trying to wrap some paper towe s around the hand of a fourth girl. The girl appeared really pale.

I joked, "I guess you don't like the sight of blood."

"No," she said, in a daze. "I really hate seeing blood."

The injured girl was a large girl, bigger than me, and much taller. I knew her fairly well; she hac been in prison for six years now. Her name was Maggie, but everyone called her Chef. She was the head cock at the prison.

She could make anything you wanted to taste good. She had taken some classes outside of prison and had done fairly well. But inside the prison, she found a passion for cooking. She was always cooking, baking, and creating some of the best-tasting food on the planet.

"Chef, are you okay though?" Glancing around the bathroom, I noticed that there was a blood on the floor and in three of the sinks.

"I think so," she said. "I just feel dizzy."

One of the girls, directly next to the sink, her name was Shandra, glanced up at me. The look on her face told me that more was going on than I knew. Her eyes and face were serious, and she was shaking her head back and forth.

I asked, "What happened?"

"I don't remember. I've been working all day and the girls told me that I cut my finger. They said it's nothing to worry about. I'm glad that you are on shift to help me. You're my favorite nurse."

Chef's knees buckled and she was helped to the floor. I stared at her hand and was surprised to see that they hadn't wrapped just one finger, but her entire hand. In fact, blood was starting to seep through the paper towels. I already had gloves on. I rushed over and grabbed a hold of the hand.

"What can you feel?" I asked.

"Not much really."

"I'm going to take a look."

Chef said, "I better be able to get stitches on this cut and be back at work tomorrow. We have a big meal planned for this holiday weekend. I've got a lot of work ahead of me."

I nodded and said, "I bet that won't be a problem...."

That was when the towels opened and the wound came into view. Blood was pouring out like a river from three or four of the fingers. It didn't take long to see that three of them had been damaged significantly, in fact, portions of the fingers were missing. There were bones sticking out from the fingers and a lot of the skin had been torn apart and was missing. I felt my stomach lurch.

I jumped into action and placed a large amount of gauze on each finger and began wrapping additional gauze rolls around the wound. I took five minutes but soon she had a club for a hand, full of gauze.

After I finished, I found that Chef was gawking at her hand. When she finally looked up at me, she said, "It doesn't look as bad as I thought. I've cut myself before, but that can easily be fixed."

I almost burst out laughing. I wasn't sure if she was joking or in shock. I decided to play along, "A quick trip to medical, and we can get this all sorted out."

I called for a wheelchair. It took a few minutes for her to get loaded on the wheelchair. I walked away and asked for an ambulance to be called. By the time we reached the outer portion of the buildings, there were a half dozen officers ready to leave the prison and the ambulance was driving into the parking lot.

Chef looked up at me and asked, "Why the ambulance?"

I said, "A hand as useful as yours, needs the most experienced attention. They will get everything sorted out."

Without another word, Chef was strapped down to a gurney and taken to a local hospital. She ended up having three or four of her fingers amputated. Two were almost completely removed.

Not long after finishing writing my nursing assessment, I returned to the kitchen and walked around. I found an industrial-sized chopper and there was a lot of blood everywhere. Several individuals were taking pictures. The found bone and tissue fragments in the machine.

Next, I went to the control room and was able to watch the video. Apparently, they had already shown in a few times by the time I arrived. I watched in horror at the screen.

Chef could be seen. She was running around the kitchen, telling everyone what to do and getting things ready. I couldn't hear what was happening, but I guess that something needed to be cut, to be added to the soup. Chef started pushing some vegetables through the machine. She worked fast and very safely. A minute or so later, the worse thing happened. Chef stepped back, ever-so-slightly, and slipped forward. Her hand was already in the machine at a safe distance. But, when she fell forward, her hand sunk into the chopper.

I turned to officer Reynolds, who happened to be standing right next to me. I said, "That seems a lot more severe than cutting a finger on a can."

Defensively he said, "I didn't see what happened. I was only reporting what I was told."

"She's lucky she didn't lose her entire hand."

Chef returned to work almost three months later. She had a lot of pain and rehab that she went through. She needed multiple surgeries to repair everything. She is getting better and better at using her affected hand. She certainly can't cut or dice like she used to be able. But she still has the mind and determination to be a great cook.

In talking with her afterward, she can't remember a single thing that happened during the injury. Shock is a crazy thing..

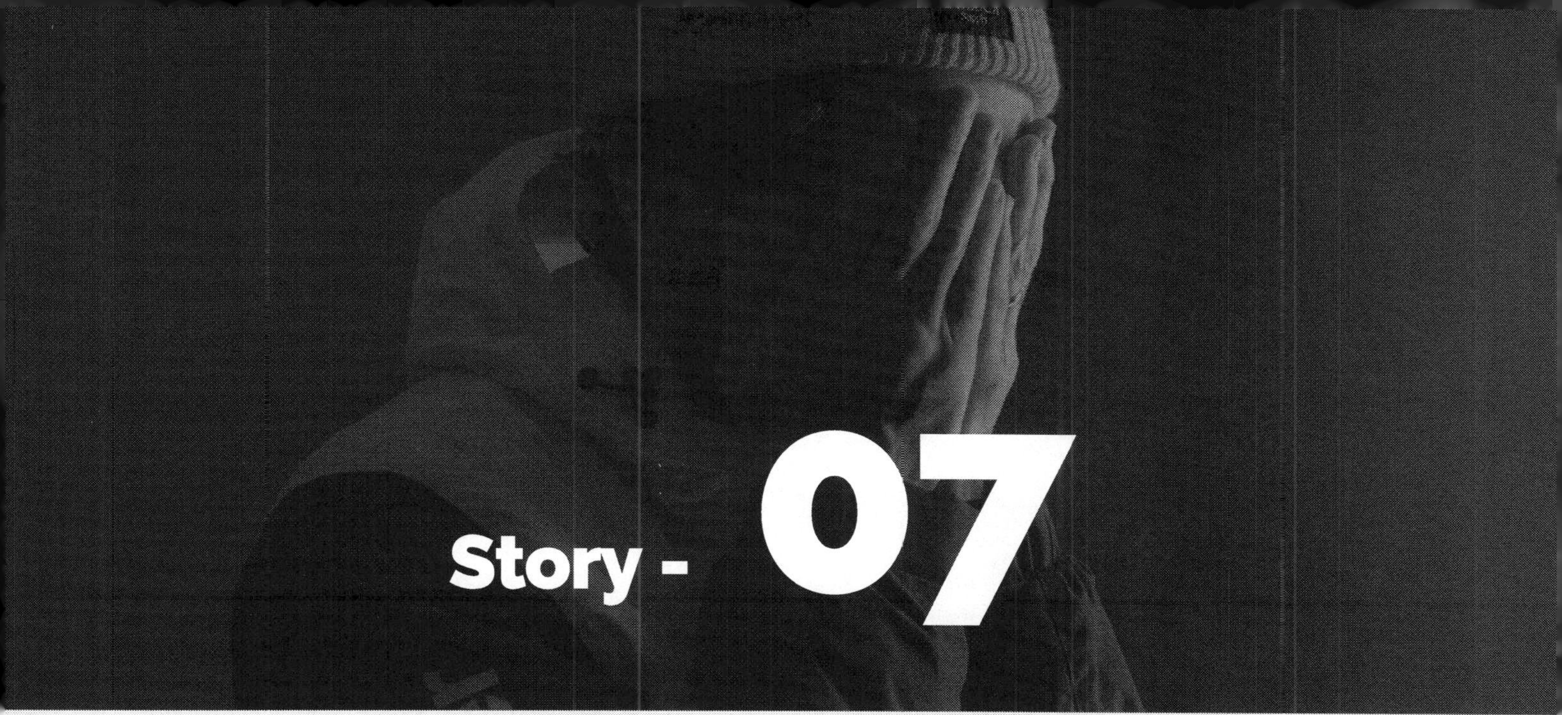

Story - 07

Any Regrets? Not at All.

My last medical appointment for the day refused to come out of his cell. He was busy watching television and told the staff that he would place another health care request to get scheduled at a later date if he felt up to it,. He told the officer specifically, "I'm here for the rest of my life. What else have I got to do?"

I quickly packed up my medical supplies and other items from the medical room. I didn't have a computer where I was working and would need to head back to the main building, to my office, to finish charting. It was getting close to the time that the tech would need to use the medical room to prepare for the afternoon med pass. Once I finished, I left the medical room and headed down a few halls towards the housing unit's front doors. Our prison has several buildings that are not attached to the main building. It wasn't but a ten-minute walk from this area across the prison grounds to my office.

The front door is used by staff and inmates going about their business inside the prison. There is a gym in another building, and much of the inmate jobs are outside of their housing unit. If the inmate is going to the rec yard, dental, to their work, classes, or any many places, they head out the front door but are still confined to the prison. As I passed several offices for the officers, I came to a section where most of the inmate's cells were located. There is a large glass area where dozens of inmates can play cards, talk, and often eat their meals. There is no chance for the inmate to escape or leave the area on their own, but they can, and do, still attempt to talk to those who pass by. I still had to cross down the hall, near the main control room, and be buzzed out the front door.

The instant some of the inmates see me, they start pestering me with questions about their medications, bottom bunk clearances, extra food, and any other medical problem they can think of at the moment. I become the most important person on the planet, for thirty seconds or less. The moment I walk out of view, they wait for the next person to pass by. This is pretty common. If I answer them, they have found a way to game the situation and potentially get something they shouldn't. There are rules for a reason. I often get asked about answering the patient's questions. It seems simple enough to just answer them in that moment, so you don't have to answer them later. Often, that can be the worst thing you can do. Except for absolute emergencies, I try to avoid these types of situations.

On this day, though, it became clear that a possible emergency was happening in the second section that I passed. I spotted a patient that was limping around the section as if injured. I first thought that he had been involved in an altercation or got injured working out, or any number of other possibilities. I knocked on the glass and waved Mr. Freeman over. Upon seeing me, he rolled his eyes, trying to ignore me. I called his name, and finally, an officer invited Mr. Freeman to come chat with me, and he was pulled out of the section.

The instant he stepped outside, Mr. Freeman said, "Look, Doctor. Good to see you and all, but I am fine. I really don't need to see you."

"I'm just making sure everything is okay. I'm not trying to harass you."

"Everything is as perfect as gold in my pocket."

I shook my head at his comparisons. I joked, "Well, I really doubt you have gold in your pocket. Does that mean things are going pretty bad?"

"It's not a crime to imagine that I have gold in my pocket. And if I did, I would be doing fantastic, just like I'm doing right now. Things couldn't be better."

"I see you are walking with a limp. Everything alright?"

"Never better."

I nodded at the officer, and Mr. Freeman was brought back into his section. Before the door closed, I said, "Let me know if you change your mind."

Mr. Freeman stuck up his middle finger and spit on the floor.

The next day, I was again scheduled in the same medical room and saw several patients with a variety of problems. Truth be told, I completely forgot about Mr. Freeman until I was walking out. I remember the encounter from yesterday and decided to try to check on him. I was astounded by how much worse he looked. He was now pale and sweating and could barely walk. His hair was a greasy mess. I learned that he had refused to eat all day. At the same time, he had a status to uphold and was walking around the section as much as possible.

I pounded on the window again, and he glanced over. He shook his head and mouthed, "Not going to talk to you today. Leave me alone." The officer passed along the information that I would be in the med central tomorrow if he needed to be seen. The next day was Saturday, and only emergent or urgent medical problems are addressed on weekends.

Med central is the prison's main area, where we keep those too sick to take care of themselves. It is also the area where the weekend (on-call) providers round on the sick patient and sees any emergencies. Partway through the next day, an emergency call was sent out, and medical was needed. Several nurses and other medical staff took a wheelchair and rushed out to a particular section. It turned out that Mr. Freeman had spent the last hour vomiting. He had refused any treatment, but medical was called when he fainted. Not long after the nurses left, Mr. Freeman was wheeled into the med central. He was awake and quite unhappy to see me. His condition had only gotten worse but was resigned to talk with me.

When I stepped into the exam room, Mr. Freeman yelled, "Doctor! You've got to help me. I'm in so much pain."

"Mr. Freeman, in order to help you, I need to know what is going on."

"If I tell you, I'm going to be in lots of trouble."

I replied, "By the way you are presenting, if you don't tell me, your life might be at risk. Your blood pressure and pulse are elevated. You have a temperature of over 101. You are sweating, and you vomited earlier. If I'm not mistaken, the tipping point was when you fainted. It looks like you already have something pretty serious going on."

"I'm not going back to the mental health unit. This was a mistake."

"I'll talk with Dr. Simmons, but I can't make any promises."

"Fine," he hissed. "The pain is driving me crazy. It's unbearable. It's the only reason I'm talking with you."

"I completely understand."

"Last week, when I was on suicide watch, I was in the old section of prison. I noticed that someone had been scraping the wall. I found a paint chip on the floor. It was as big as my thumbnail and thick."

"I'm guessing that you didn't turn that in."

"No way. I had spent the entire time wondering how my insides would look."

"Like your stomach?"

"And more." Mr. Freeman suddenly appeared as if he was transfixed, seeing something no one else could see."

I really didn't like where this conversation was going. I've learned that if you react, the inmates will often close down. You have to pretend that what they said means nothing. Trying to sound calm, I said, "Keep going."

"I snuck the paint chip in my bum hole and brought it back to my cell."

"That sounds painful."

"It wasn't too bad."

"Does your rectum hurt now?"

"Not at all."

"Continue."

"I hid the paint chip in my cell. A few days later, at night, I started thinking about my insides again. I just couldn't get it out of my mind. That's when I pulled out the paint chip and started to explore. You know, I've always been very curious about my penis. I started cutting the sac below my penis. It didn't bleed nearly as much as I thought."

Still trying to remain calm, I asked, "Was it painful?"

"Not at all."

"How much did you cut?"

"As much as I could. It was only a few inches, I think. I put my fingers in a few times. It didn't turn out as cool as I thought it would be."

"Did you cut anywhere else?"

"Nope."

"When did it start hurting?"

"Well. The next day, I had another great idea. I started shoving things into the new hole."

"Um...what?"

"I had some leftover lunch and a Styrofoam cup, and several other small items. I pushed as much as I could into the hole. At first, it felt really weird to have my sac so big. A few days later, that's when it started hurting."

"Is all that material still inside the hole?"

"Yes. The skin started to get red, and there was some swelling. I think that this morning there was some drainage." He laughed awkwardly. "But truthfully, if it weren't for this pain, I wouldn't have come to talk with you. It's the worst pain I've ever felt."

I mumbled, "Can't imagine." I felt my stomach turn, and I was suddenly nauseous. I pushed forward and added, "Unfortunately, it sounds like you have an infection. We can't stop the pain unless we remove that material. It is what is causing you to be sick. Are you okay if I take a look and start cleaning out the area?"

The next few hours were some of the most difficult in my time at the Prison. Cutting open the area and removing the material and infection was overwhelming. He was in substantial pain. The amount of swelling and redness is hard to describe. Turned out, the scrotum affected was about the size of a volleyball. There was so much material that we filled a small pink basin. He had food, Styrofoam, plastic, wood chips, and other items. Once all the material was removed, the area was cleaned, and a huge dressing was placed over the area.

He was admitted to med central and monitored over the next several days and was on heavy antibiotics and pain medication. He was also given a fair amount of mental health medications. It took him weeks and weeks to heal. He had to meet with mental health a few times a day to make sure that he didn't try to harm himself again. Three months later, the wound finally closed, and it appeared as normal as possible. A scar formed, and the scrotum remained slightly larger than the other side.

At our last visit prior to being discharged from med central, I asked, "Any regrets about doing this to yourself?"

"Not at all."

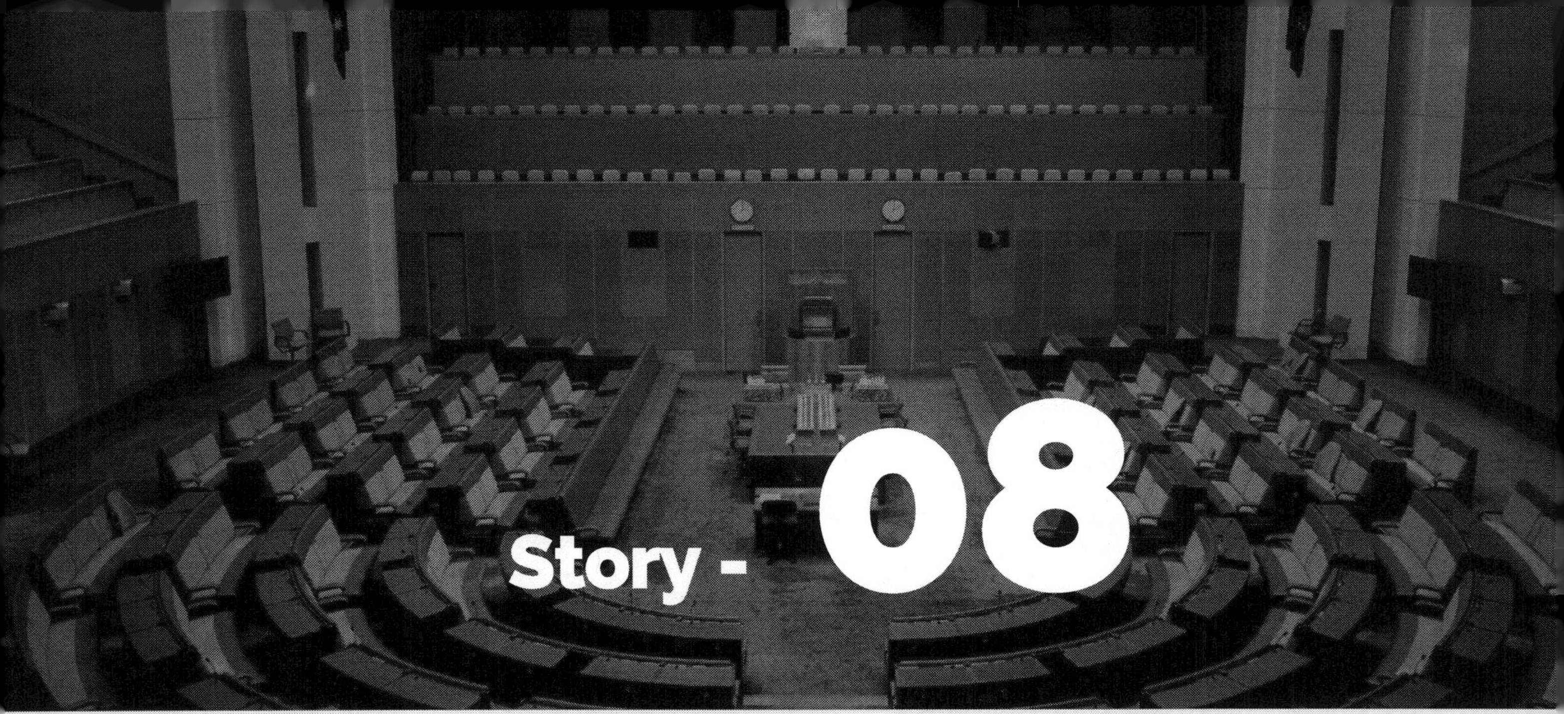

Strangling Someone in the Courtroom

A nurse practitioner (APRN) was called to some court proceeding about a patient refusing to restart his mental health medications. The patient had been in and out of jail, and Ryle had seen him several times. In fact, she had seen him have a significant improvement to his mental health and overall health while in jail when he was willing to be on his medications. The problem was that Mr. Beckendorf had been refusing to take his medications for the last few months. This had eventually got him in trouble and landed him in this courtroom. The judge wanted to get her input on how well medications had worked inside the jail and if this patient really needed to be court-ordered to take his mental health medications and attend services provided by the local mental health group.

Forcing a patient to take medications can be a tricky thing. Often it needs to be court-approved whether this is inside the jail or outside; you really have to provide a need to force medications. Often there are a few hearings, and mental health specialists are contacted, and evaluations are done.

Ryle arrived early to the courtroom and had many of her notes. She had reviewed the patient and the medications that he'd been on in the past. She waited for an hour before the court opened, and she was called into the courtroom. The judge was just getting back from a break. Simultaneously, as the judge was coming into the courtroom, Mr. Beckendorf was also being escorted into the courtroom.

Mr. Beckendorf was a middle-aged man who wore clothes that hadn't been washed in months or years. His hair hadn't been cut since he was released from jail two months ago. Ryle anticipated how he might smell, act, and she was worr ed about possible yelling and screaming that Mr. Beckendorf might do. He appeared quite unstable. She knew that at times, Mr. Beckendorf could get angry and violent, and she was hoping that wouldn't happen today. Over the last two months, he had been brought to the jail countless times but released the same day. He would be given a few hours to sober and get his fingerprints, and then he was free to leave the jail.

Mr. Beckendorf's problems became more apparent when he decided to make his home, the bathroom at the local McDonalds. One night, a week ago, he snuck into the McDonalds before it closed and found a way to evade the workers before they locked up for the night. He had helped himself to some of the food in the kitchen area and had dragged some boxes and other items to the women's bathroom, and created his own bedroom. The next day, when the employees arrived, the bathroom door was locked, and despite using the key, they couldn't find a way to get it open. Around noon, the police were called, and it took a few hours before they convinced Mr. Beckendorf to open the doors. I think he was starting to get hungry again. Mr. Beckendorf has an extensive criminal history and mental health history. However, at times, he denies both, which leads him to refuse his medications.

Earlier this year, while he was in jail, he was restarted on mediations. It had taken a month to convince him to allow Ryle to start him on these new medications. In a matter of weeks, he was doing so much better. In fact, it was the best that Ryle had ever seen him. During that jail stay, he would wash daily, eat regularly, and take his medications. This is often what the medical staff in prisons and jails see, patients are better when they take their medications, and sometimes it takes going to jail to get the help they need. Once they are released, however, some patients stop taking their medications.

Mr. Beckendorf was eventually released, and it didn't take him long to stop picking up his medications and attending his meetings. He often thought he didn't need them, or alcohol or meth was far better for him. Hence, why Ryle was seeing the judge today. Since the McDonald's incident, he was refusing to talk to anyone in mental health. He was on the verge of returning to jail for an extended period of time.

Ryle waited until it was her turn to address the judge. Several other people had given their opinions and other thoughts. As Ryle approached the podium, she noticed that Mr. Beckendorf appeared confused and mentally unstable, even worse than when she first saw him. Before she reached the podium, Mr. Beckendorf stood and began inching himself away from his seat. At first, no one else saw what was happening. Ryle stopped and watched Mr. Beckendorf, fearing that he would run away or even towards her or the judge.

He continued backing up towards the sidewall and slid into a small gap between two pillars. There was still enough room to see what was going on. Soon, the judge, other lawyers, and everyone else in the courtroom noticed that Ryle had stopped walking. All eyes focused on where she was looking. Mr. Beckendorf was suddenly very mad and began screaming. At first, it was impossible to understand what he was saying. It was apparent that he didn't see the world as Ryle or the others were seeing it.

Mr. Beckendorf screamed, "Why would I ever think of going there with you?"

Mr. Beckendorf was quiet for a moment, and Ryle realized that he was listening to a conversation with an imaginary person.

He continued, his voice almost shouting, "Like your beauty could ever deceive me enough to believe that."

Another pause.

"I'm not going to get naked here for you."

Another pause

"Get out of my sight. Don't ever let me catch you here again. You better believe you will pay the ultimate price."

Each of the phrases was screamed at increasingly higher pitches and with more and more anger. Ryle watched Mr. Beckendorf flinch like he'd been hit with a sledgehammer. Mr. Beckendorf reacted in such a way that Ryle would never forget. He turned to his side, facing the back of the courtroom, and lifted both hands, and began strangling, very violently, the imaginary person he was talking with. It was not a few seconds but over and over again. Foul language surrounded by the words, "Die," and "Die," were heard by the entire courtroom.

Ryle barely had to say anything to the judge. The visual evidence was obvious enough. Mr. Beckendorf was committed to the jail the same day, and it took less than two weeks for him to be transferred to the state hospital the same day. He has been there for over one year now. Ryle has a sinking suspicion that she might see Mr. Beckendorf again one day back in jail. Someone rarely stays in the state hospital indefinitely. Hopefully, the next time she sees him, he will have remained on his medications.

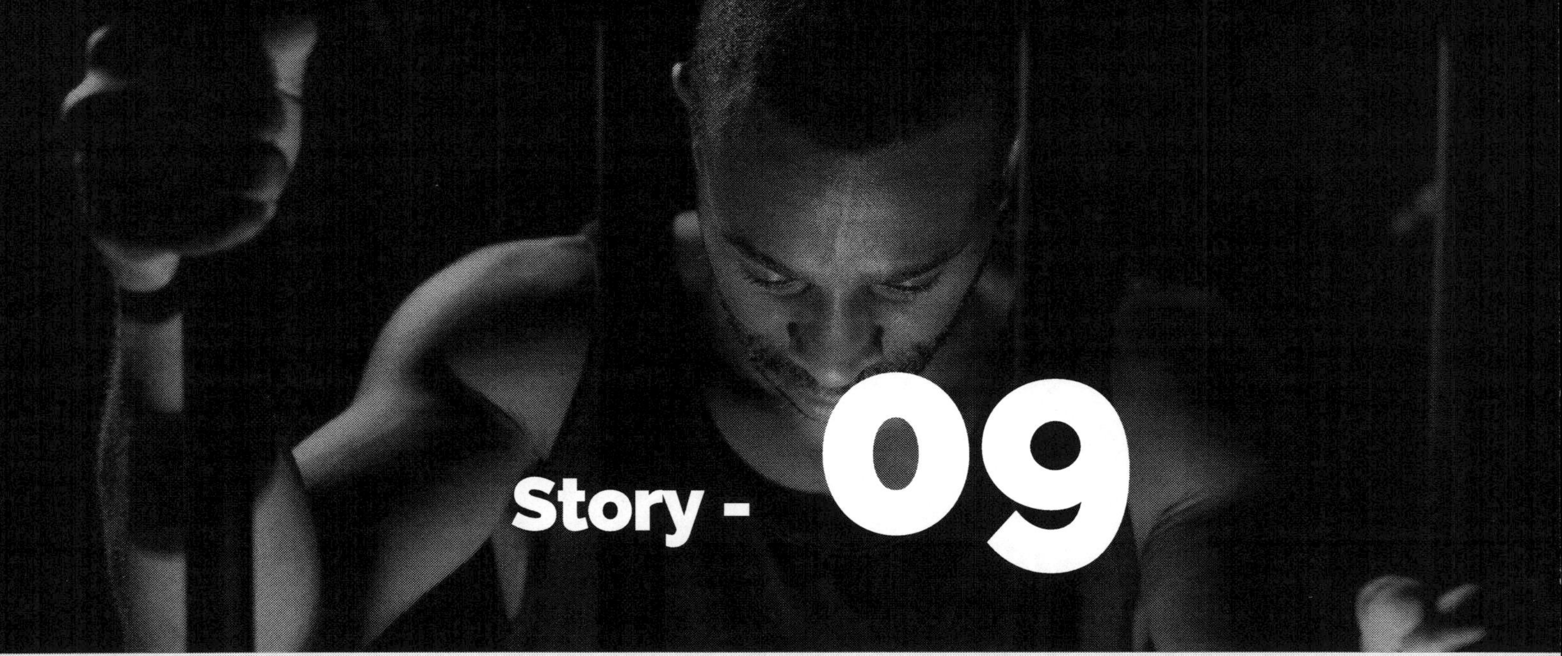

Story - 09

When Skin Turns Black, In A Very Unexpected Area

Often, if there is a medical emergency, I am notified over the radio and asked to head out to a certain area of the jail. I usually bring the necessary supplies that are needed if I know what is going on. However, on this day, there was radio silence, and instead, the officer brought a traumatic looking patient to the medical room for an assessment. This was the moment I found out about the potential emergency.

Jared, the officer said, “Inmate Omari reported an unsettling problem. I felt that he needed a little privacy to see what is going on. Nurse Jamie, I’m so happy that you’re still here. Would you mind taking a look?”

“What seems to be the problem?”

“Um,” Inmate Omari hesitated. “My balls are turning black.”

The patient, an inmate who had been at the jail for a few years, had never really made a medical complaint in the two and a half years that he had been here.

"When did this start?" I asked.

"Six of seven days ago."

"How come you didn't tell us sooner? Did you turn in a health care request (HCR)?"

"My cellmate said that it would go away. I showed him, and he says that this is common. He told me that he was a nurse outside of jail. When it didn't go away, I called over Officer Perriman."

Shaking my head, I said, "Your cellmate wasn't a nurse, and this isn't a common problem. But I'll need to take a look to really understand what is going on."

"I don't believe you. My roommate said it's just a rash."

"How about we take a look and find out what it really going on."

"I guess that would be fine," said Inmate Omari. "But I don't want a girl looking at my junk."

"Officer Perriman will be here as well. Nothing to be embarrassed about."

Rashes are some of the most common complaints inside jails and prisons. Everyone thinks that everything is a rash. Most of the time, it is not a big deal. It also seems that unpredictable rashes happen only in jail. A patient might be fine outside of jail, but inside they have a reoccurring rash that never goes away.

The assessment was done quickly and effectively. The shock of what I saw was surprising. Inmate Omari did not have a rash, but something much more concerning. Sometimes, patients embellish their symptoms. This patient was not. Both of his testicles looked like black marbles. I asked that the patient wait outside of the medical office as I called the jail provider, a local provider.

When he answered, I said, "Doctor Jeong, we've got a pretty serious problem at the jail."

Doctor Jeong said, "What kind of a problem are we talking about?"

"Inmate Omari, who came in a few months ago, is having skin problems. The color of the skin of both testicles is black. He states the problem has been going on for several days and reported it to his cellmate. It hasn't gotten any better, and he reported it to Officer Periman today. He was just brought down to the med room.

"Does it look like a bruise? Could he have gotten injured?"

"It doesn't look like a bruise. It looks pretty bad."

"Both testicles?"

"Yes." She cringed. "The skin looks sort of wet and gross."

"Could it be an infection?" Doctor Jeong asked. "Do you see any drainage?"

"No. It's like the entire skin is moist, and there is some skin breakdown, especially on the lower part of the testicles, closer to the legs."

"How are the patient's vitals?"

"He has a temperature, and his blood pressure and heart rate are slightly elevated."

"Okay," he paused for a moment. "It does sound like a possible infection."

"Also," the nurse said. "Not sure how to say this, but both testicles are cold to the touch."

"Can you send a picture?"

"Sure."

The picture was sent, and Doctor Jeong was able to review the picture. It didn't take long for him to call back. Speaking with Nurse Jamie, he said, "I think that we are looking at gangrene of both testicles. This is a pretty serious emergency. How long did you say this has been going on?"

Nurse Jaime said, "I guess he was super embarrassed at what was happening and didn't want to tell anyone at first. He told his roommate, who convinced him that it wasn't a big deal. He says it has been going on for more than a week and getting worse."

"How long would it take for an ambulance to get there and take him to the local hospital?"

"About two hours."

"Can the local hospital do surgery, if necessary?"

"I doubt it. Not this specialized. They'll probably have to take him into the city."

"That will add another few hours. We need a better option. I'll call you back."

Twenty-five minutes later, Doctor Jeung called back with updated information. "I've talked with the sheriff and the local authorities. The only option will be for a small airplane to fly to the local airfield. The jail will transport the patient to the airfield, and an officer will accompany the patient to the hospital. The flight to the city will be thirty minutes, and there will be an ambulance waiting at the airfield. I've also contacted the hospital, sent them pictures, and they will be ready to receive the patient. A surgical group will be ready if surgery is indeed warranted."

Nurse Jamie set off and prepared the inmate for the transfer. He had to have shackles placed around his waist and legs. His hands were attached to the shackles around his waist. The ride to the local airport was extremely uncomfortable.

As they went over another bump, Inmate Omari said, "This is torture. This is, by far, the worst pain I've ever had. Make it stop!"

Officer Dickerson, the transportation officer, said, "The nurse said that you might have an infection. Once you get to the hospital, they will take care of you."

"Can't they just give me some antibiotics back at the jail? This is way too painful."

"I am pretty sure that if they could keep you at the jail, they would have. This might be a little more complicated."

Inmate Omari and Officer Dickerson arrived at the local airport and found a small plane waiting for them. Both of them boarded the plane, and it took off. The ride in the airplane was only moderately less painful than the van ride.

As the plane landed, Inmate Omari started having cold sweats and began feeling nauseous. The ambulance quickly strapped Omari to a gurney, and along with Officer Dickerson, they were sped off to the city hospital.

The examination at the hospital was quick. Doctor Samuels agreed with the initial diagnosis of gangrene, and he felt that surgery was needed for debridement or removal of some of the skin.

Dr. Sameuls spoke with Inmate Omari to explain things. "Do you know what gangrene is?"

"I think I've heard of it before."

"It is when there is the death of body tissue due to either a lack of blood flow or a serious bacterial infection. Often, we see gangrene in toes, fingers, feet, and other parts of the body. It is quite rare to have this in the testicles."

"If it is an infection," Inmate Omari asked, "can I be okay with just antibiotics. Maybe IV antibiotics?"

"Unfortunately not. This is serious. In fact, there is tissue death in this case. Surgery will be needed to remove the tissue."

"How much tissue will need to be removed?"

"I won't know until I see how things are during surgery."

Inmate Omari said, "If that's the only option, let's get this done."

Doctor Samuels said, "Let's get you prepped for surgery."

Several hours later, Doctor Samuels returned to the recovery room. Inmate Omari was less groggy than half an hour ago. Dr. Samuels said, "Well, the severity of the gangrene was more than we thought."

"What does that mean?" Inmate Omari asked.

"The testicles are part of the male reproductive system. The sac that protects the testicles is called the scrotum. The scrotum is the tissue where the gangrene was located. We had to remove all of the skin associated with the scrotum."

"Are you kidding me? What happened to my testicles?"

"That is the interesting part. We were able to save the testicles. You can still have children in the future if you want."

"So, where are my testicles?"

"We had to cut open the inside of both of your legs. There was plenty of tissue available. Essentially, you have a testicle in your inner thigh."

"Oh, my word," Omari said. "How is that possible?"

"This was a really bad situation, but we made a good decision and found a way for this to work."

Inmate Omari asked, "Are they going to be in my legs forever?"

"Not necessarily. A few months after surgery, we will explore some different options."

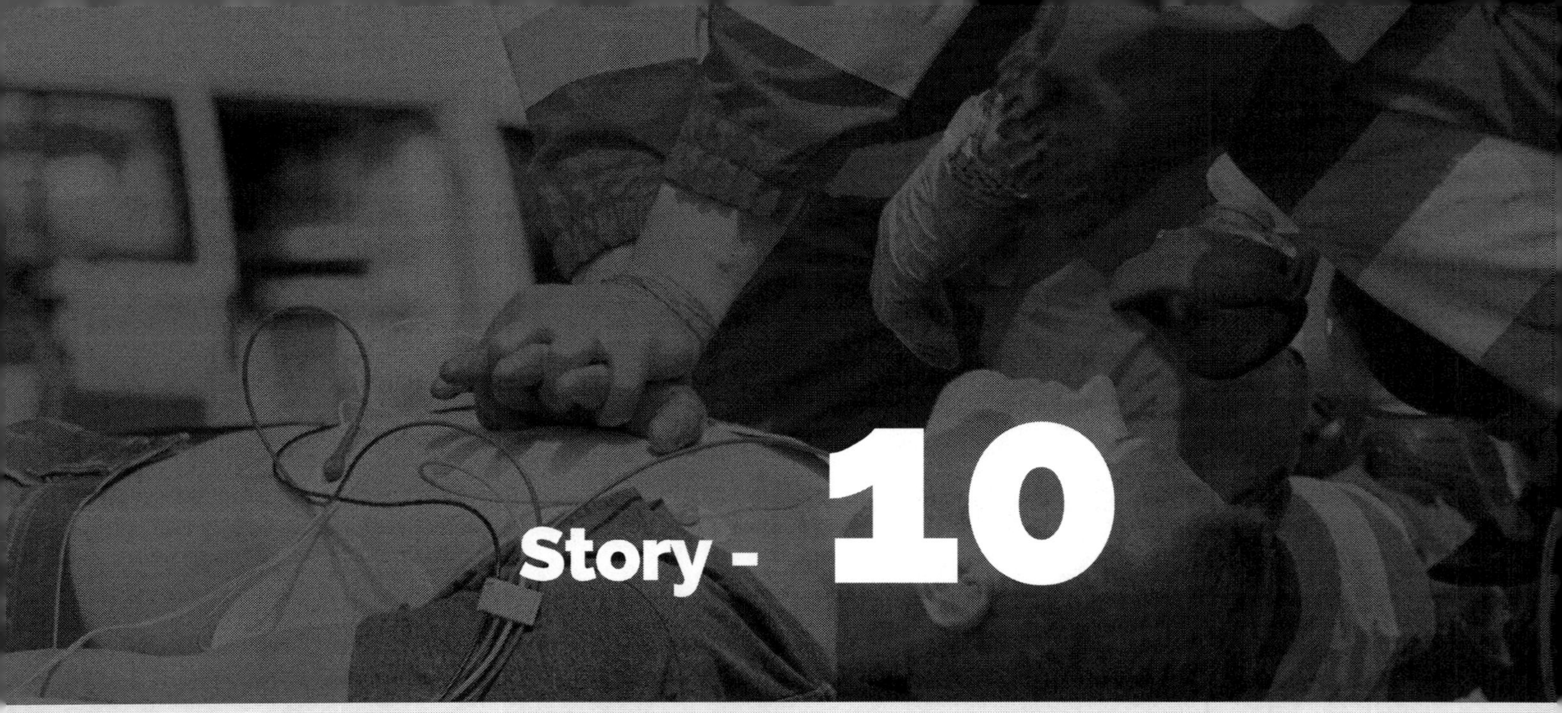

Aftermath of a Prison Fight, Two Unconscious and Blood Everywhere

A shy inmate was informed that he would be moving to a new section of the prison, in fact, into a different building. He had only been in prison for a few months, and this move wasn't unexpected. The intake process had been the first sixty days that he had been in prison. He had been bunked with several inmates over that time; all had been new inmates to the correctional setting. Together they had gone through the orientation process as well as the intake medical and mental health screenings. This inmate had also had his teeth cleaned for the first time in his life.

He felt pretty anxious over the last week when he was told about his pending move. The first move is the big one. It will often define your time in prison. Your first cellmate will help you navigate the tougher aspects of prison. They will help you understand who to be friends with and who to ignore, where he was allowed to go and what was off-limits. As Gustavo left those he met, he wondered how different they might be when he saw them again. Prison changes you. As Gustavo stepped into his new cell, he knew instantly that this was not going to be a good transition on his part.

The cell was perfectly clean. There was a sparkle on the floor that was impossible to find in any other section of the prison. The prison wasn't old, but it had seen its fair share of problems. The cell was a typical two-man cell with a bunk bed in the right-hand corner. The toilet and sink were just the left. Further back on the left was a small table built into the wall.

The deep voice that sprung from the shadows made Gustavo's knees shake. "You my new cellie?"

"Sure am."

A figure stepped into view. The tall man was ten years older than Gustavo was. His face was tight, and it was obvious he had been in several fights. He was big and had plenty of muscles. The eyes were the most concerning. They were blank, almost as if he didn't really care what happened. The man said, "I'm Rip."

"Hello. I'm Gustavo." He put his hand out to shake and continued, "I've been locked down for two months. I'm..."

Rip knocked his hand away. "I don't care who you are or how long you've been here. There are a few rules in my house. I own everything in this section and this cell."

Trying to act brave, Gustavo said, "Which bed is mine?"

"Not in this house. You cannot eat, breathe, or piss unless I say it's alright. You will rent your bed from me, and it will cost you."

Gustavo shuddered. "What's the cost?"

"This room will stay clean. You will wash anything I ask. If I want you to hide something, you will. You'll be the lookout for the guards. You do exactly what I say when I say it."

"I can do that." At that moment, Gustavo thought he was going to be sick. He glanced at the toilet. Rip noticed.

Rip hissed, "For one week, you cannot use that toilet."

"Where else am I supposed to go?"

"Not my problem."

Gustavo worked hard for the next three days and two nights. He cleaned and hustled and did whatever was told of him, just like a dog. In fact, that became his nickname. All of Rip's friends and other inmates around the section would say, "Hey, dog this...." and "Hey, dog that..." It was downright embarrassing. Gustavo ate none of his own trays and was forced to purchase $50 of commissary for Rip and his friends.

Rip did 300 or more pushups every day. He worked out for six hours or more. Gustavo brought water and other food. Rip slept when he wanted and did what he wanted - within the boundaries of the prison. Gustavo watched, and it was clear that Rip was, in fact, the leader of this section of the prison. He told pretty much everyone what to do. To Gustavo, it seemed that even some of the prison guards feared Rip. Gustavo had never seen anything like it.

By the third night, things had gone from bad to worse for Gustavo. He was suffering through all the chores, cleaning, and other errands he had been given. Some of them were downright embarrassing. He was only allowed to sleep for two hours each of the first two nights. He was tired and angry. But more importantly, he really had to go to the bathroom. It was nearing midnight, and Rip gave him four hours to sleep. He lay down and instantly fell to sleep. Two hours later, though, he woke, and using the bathroom was now, an emergency. He didn't have a choice. Rip was asleep in the bunk below him.

Gustavo snuck down silently to the floor. He tiptoed across to the bathroom. There was minimal privacy when using the toilet in prison, and this cell was no different. Fear coursed through him, but he also knew that he was going to go to the bathroom one way or another. His body could no longer hold it.

As he sat down, relief flooded through him. Just as the last amount had left him, a voice said, "What the hell do you think you are doing?"

A fight ensued, and a short time later, the prison's medical staff and several officers were called to see the aftermath. When they arrived on the scene, there was blood everywhere. Officers were unsure of what to do because it appeared that both individuals were injured. There were several nurses and a few CNAs that arrived. The first inmate was lying on the floor near the toilet. He had been hit so many times, his face was swollen, and there was blood pooling on the floor. The second was lying on the floor near the center of the room. It seemed that this inmate had fewer injuries, but he was unconscious on the floor.

Quickly the cell became secure by the officers. Three nurses began treating the first patient. His arm had been broken, and his head was gashed open. His face was so swollen that his eyes were shut. He had been sprawled next to the toilet and against the wall. It was impossible to understand how he had been found n that position, and took a few minutes to pull him out from where he had fallen.

I was one of the nurses that attended to the first patient. He was barely breathing. I asked, "What happened?"

Officer Davenport, assisting on the scene, said, "This is Ricardo and Gustavo. Most people call Ricardo -Rip. I thought these guys were getting along. There was nothing leading up to this point. About thirty minutes ago, things changed. I heard screaming and hollering and a whole bunch of fighting. The entire section was woken up."

"Which is which?"

"Rip is by the toilet, and Gustavo is back there on the floor."

"Rip is huge. What happened here?"

"The other inmates say that Gustavo started hitting Rip and wouldn't stop."

Additional nurses entered the cell and began attending to Gustavo. Smelling salt was used, and a few minutes later, he was able to sit up and answer a few questions. He was hurting in his arms, legs, and back of the head. A quick exam showed that he had minimal injuries. A few minutes later, he began crying.

Rip, on the other hand, was severely beaten, and he stayed unconscious despite the smelling salts. An ambulance was called. The patient was cared for by several of the medical staff. He was placed on a backboard, an IV was placed, moved to a gurney. Several other emergency treatments were done to help the head wound, broken arm, and such. The ambulance arrived within minutes, and Rip was transported to the hospital in bad shape.

Gustavo was transported to the medical unit. In our facility, there is a central medical unit on the bottom floor of the main building with approximately fifteen to twenty medical beds and another twenty mental health beds. This particular section of the prison wasn't connected with the main building. The patient was loaded in a van and transported to the medical unit. One of our providers was waiting for Gustavo. He ended up having a concussion and needed several staples in the back of his head. He had some scratch marks on his arms, but most everything else was normal.

Investigations came in while things were finishing. They listened, without words, to Gustavo's side of the story.

He said, "Rip attacked me while I was sitting on the toilet. I was able to jump out of the way, and he just missed me. He crashed into the toilet, and I started hitting him. I hit him with the metal toilet seat, my fists, and anything I could. He fought back and hit me a few times. I must've stumbled back and fallen and hit my head. You must understand that he had already attacked me several times, and he has done terrible things. I wasn't allowed to leave the cell without his permission. He was keeping me hostage. He had tons of friends too. He was refusing to allow me to use the toilet. I had to go so bad that I snuck down in the middle of the night. He attacked, and I snapped. I feel bad about what happened, but I didn't have another choice."

Rip survived and returned to prison about two months later. His head wound was severe, and he lost the ability of some movement on the left side of his body, similar to a stroke. He went to a special housing unit for those with severe medical and mental limitations. Gustavo had several interdisciplinary meetings, as well as court proceedings. There was no one who was willing to testify to what really happened. It turned out to be

Gustavo's word, and that wasn't good enough. In the end, ten years were added to his sentence. As a side note, all toilet seats in prison were removed.

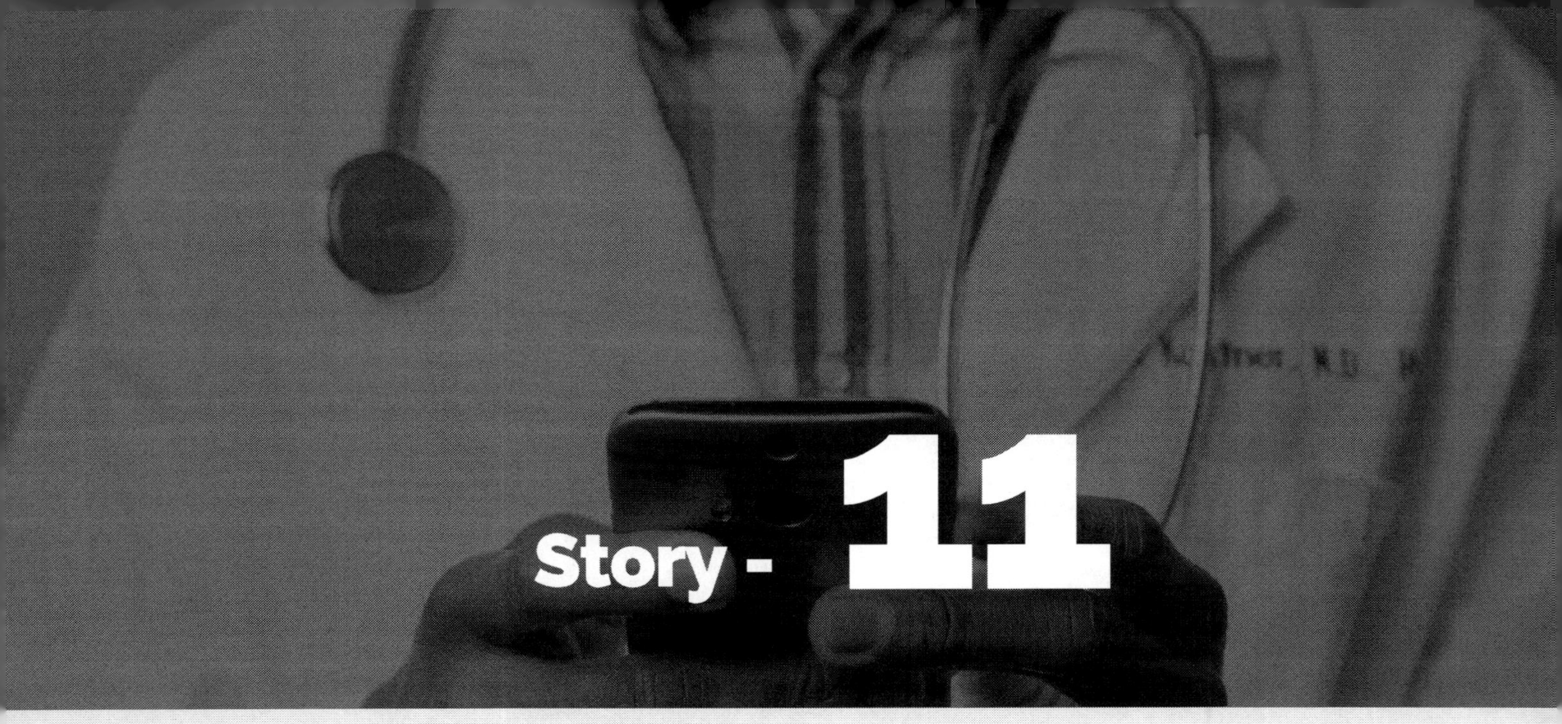

Story - 11

A Crazy Mixture of a Riot and a Medical Emergency

Riots are an uncommon thing to happen in most prisons. A select few prisons have seen a larger number of episodes of absolute disorder and chaos by certain groups or individuals. Riots can have devastating consequences and often lead to staff and inmate injuries, lockdowns, violence, and retaliation. Causes of riots can vary from anger at prison staff, gang violence, boredom, and many more. Whatever the reason, riots become much more effective when there are more inmates involved and/or with better detailed planning.

Such a riot occurred in our prison several years ago. We had heard some of the inmates' grumblings and knew that they were upset about how cold the prison was at night. We have an older prison, and it is harder to heat the entire building. One specific area seems to have a more challenging time controlling the temperature. Common sense, from an outside perspective, would be to give out more blankets. But truthfully, that gives the inmates more weapons and opportunities to hurt themselves or others. We had seen similar problems five years earlier when we had an even colder spell.

Four days after Christmas, a few years back, we had a riot that started around seven in the evening. Cell blocks in this particular area are divide into 4 sections. Each section had 15 cells on the bottom floor and 15 cells on the top floor. There are typically 56-60 inmates in each section. That means - this building holds at most 224-230 inmates. The section that started the riot was #4. There were typically officers in each section that monitor inmates, solve problems, watch and prevent problems, and much more. Sometimes they had to leave a section for one reason or another. They are always coming in and out of a particular section. There was also a control room that monitors each section, unlocks doors, and communicates with other areas of the prison. Luckily, during this riot, the officer was dealing with something else, in another area, when it started.

Approximately ten of the cells on the bottom floor rushed out with their mattresses and created a barrier. There were approximately twenty inmates that were doing this. One of the first steps in a riot is to create a barrier for when the officers start sending in pepper spray, and this prevents the officers from seeing what was happening behind the barrier. Pepper spray comes in different forms. Sprays and pepper balls were often used. There are foggers, but we didn't have one of these at the time. Another dozen or so inmates started pasting newspaper and other papers to the lower edge of the section wall. Looking into the section from the control room or a hallway is done through specialized plexiglass. It is a wide-open area, and therefore, the inmates were attempting to reduce the visibility quickly.

It didn't take long for the staff to realize what was happening. Other officers were called, along with the medical staff and administration. Soon many people were mobilizing and coming to this area of the prison. Several specialized teams were created to attempt to solve this problem peacefully.

It quickly became apparent that no demands were going to be given early on. Many staff began speculating about the reasons for the riot. Escape was not really a possibility, but suddenly items were smashed into the section's outer walls. These were beds or other larger items. They were attempting to destroy whatever they could. Destruction and riot are almost always used together.

Pepper spray was soon deployed into this section. The inmates were well prepared with torn shirts and towels draped over their mouths and soaked in water. If things got too bad, an individual would retreat into some of the upper rooms where they would open the window an inch or so. Bars prevented any type of escape. Fans pushed around the air. Soon, a cloud hung over the entire section. However, the inmates did not seem to be giving up anytime soon. In one or two of the back rooms, it appeared that the inmates were trying to light fires.

An hour or two into the riot, the entire lower area of the plexiglass was covered with newspaper or other papers. This made looking into the area more difficult. The inmates were also trying to throw things at the cameras inside the section. A few had been knocked out of place. Ladders were brought in by the officers to get a higher vantage point and a better look. When the first officer climbed the ladder, he noticed that at least 30 inmates were attempting to damage the bottom floor. There were piles of mattresses that were carefully arranged, and inmates were assigned to hold them up. Indeed, two fires had been started.

It was decided that a paintball gun would be used to spray pepper spray in the back regions of the section. These balls were often used to spray pepper chemicals for further distances. When the balls break, the chemical was released. A small hole cut in the upper portion of the wall is opened, and the same officer began shooting into the section. Again, the inmates were ready for this, and the mattresses were placed in position, some of them lifted off the ground. The pepper balls smack into the mattresses harmlessly. It was clear that some of the balls didn't break. These were gathered by the inmates. Tactics were changed, and instead, the balls were shot into the cement and off the walls, spraying the chemicals around the room.

A second hole is opened, and from a different angle, the room was resprayed. The leader of the riot was targeted. He had wrapped a towel around his head. He had removed his shirt and pants and was wearing shorts. The temperature inside the section had increased substantially. It was easy to pick him out as he was screaming and shouting and willing others to stay strong. His voice was heard above all the others. More items were being brought out of cells. A cluster of people took had removed one of the cell's doors. They were moving it towards the front to use it as a battering ram. One of the officers shot pepper spray in their direction. The closer they get to the front of the section, the harder it is to spray them.

The leader bellowed and ran, back and forth, behind the mattress wall as several more pepper balls were sent in his direction. It was almost like a Braveheart moment. On his third pass, he suddenly stopped screaming and fell to the floor. He was running so quickly that he slid several feet. Just as soon as his screams stop, they restart, but this time, they were screams of pure agony. Everything in the section stops, including those hammering the walls with the door. Inmates began spilling out of their cells to look at what was happening.

Less than five minutes later, the riot had completely ended. Most of the inmates were sent to the upper rooms. Once the inmates were secured, several officers rush into the section, put out fires, remove newspapers from the walls, and took control of the situation. Our medical staff hurried into the area and immediately began to administer medical help to the riot leader and several others who had been injured or were having trouble with the smoke and/or pepper spray.

The entire time, the leader had been screaming nonstop. He was pleading for the other inmates to stop what they were doing so that he could get medical help. It worked.

Officers quickly handcuffed the inmate to prevent further problems.

The first nurse, Vincent, arrived near the inmate and asked, "What hurts? Are you having trouble breathing?"

Inmate Bertrand yelled, "Get me out of here!"

Vincent replied, "Tell me what is going on."

"Not here."

"Can you stand?"

"I can't walk. It hurts so bad." Inmate Bertrand demanded, "Get me on a gurney and get me out of here."

The gurney was brought in, and Inmate Bertrand was quickly transported to the medical department.

The other inmates were quickly removed from this section. Ten of them had severe breathing issues and needed to be closely monitored. Showers, new clothing, and lockdown cells were given to each inmate involved in the riot. There had been a dozen fights between inmates and more damage than you could imagine. Turns out, there were about fifteen inmates that played no part in the riot.

It didn't take long for inmate Bertrand to arrive in medial. He was screaming the entire time he was transported. Much of what he said was unrecognizable. A doctor was waiting for Inmate Bertrand to arrive. Doctor Yapp asked, "How is he?"

Nurse Vincent said, "He won't stop screaming."

Bertrand was moved into an examination room. Two officers stay close by as Doctor Yapp, Nurse Vincent, and two other medical staff tended to the inmate.

Finally, Inmate Bertrand said something that they could understand, "My balls! My balls!"

They removed his shorts and underwear and found an explosion of pepper spray residue entering the room. Everyone began coughing immediately. Masks were passed out, and all the clothes were removed from the room. Between burning eyes, Doctor Yapp found that a pepper ball had directly hit one of Inmate Bertrand's testicles. It had damaged the skin and the tissue significantly. A short time later, Inmate Bertrand began vomiting either from pain or the pepper spray, but most likely both.

The scrotal damage turned out to be a medical emergency. Inmate Bertrand was transported to the local hospital and quickly into surgery. The affected testicle was removed. From that time forward, Inmate Bertrand never caused a single problem inside the prison again.

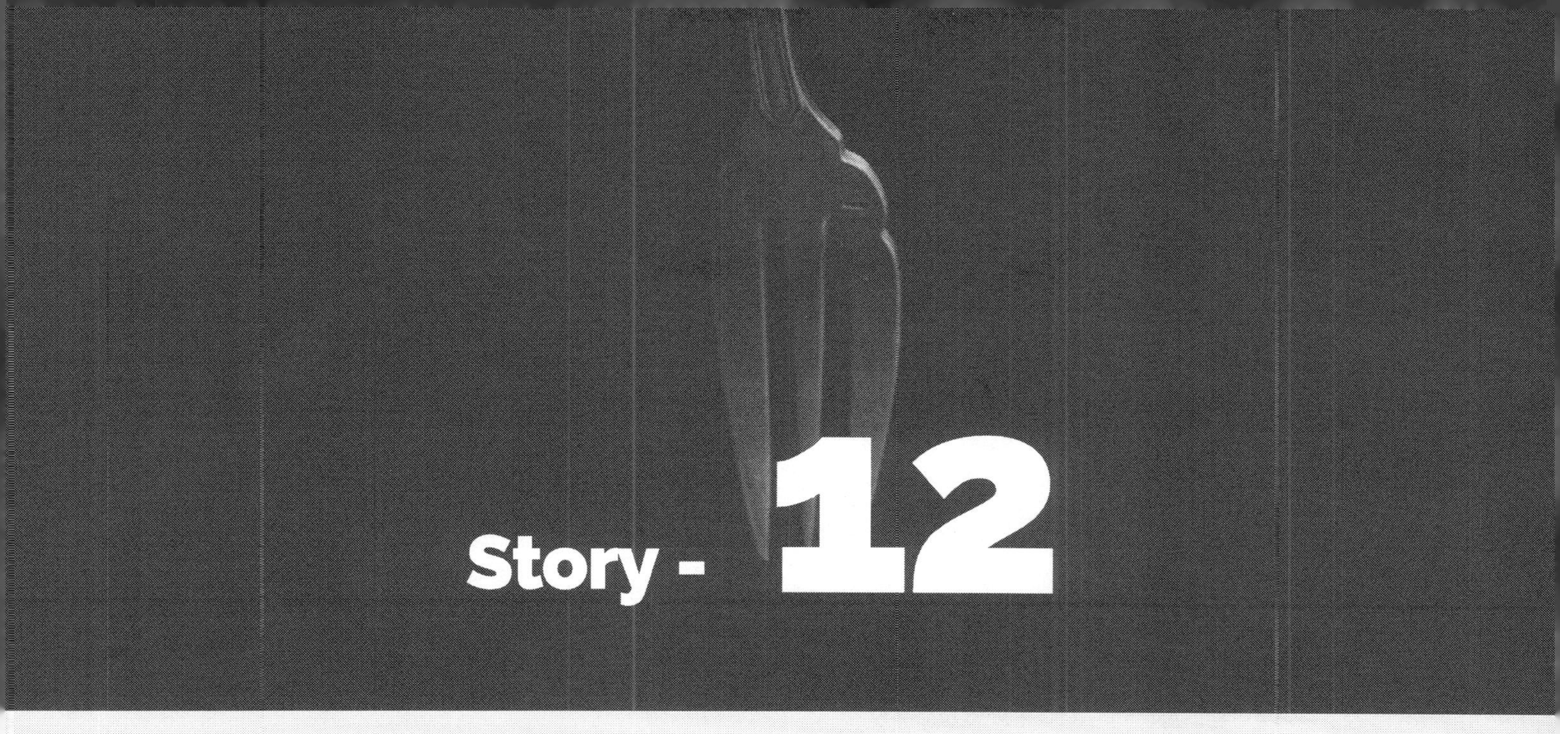

Story - 12

Complications From a Hunger Strike

Whether you believe it to be a good thing or not, inmates have legal rights. Some of those legal rights include refusing to eat, drink, take life-saving medications, and many more. Medical personnel in prisons and jails can't force inmates to take their medication or allow a necessary medical procedures. Sometimes, the court system, mental health professionals, lawyers, and judges can intervene to force a medication and/or a treatment. This is a complicated process and is often a lengthy one as well. Several different mental health evaluations and such are involved along with court proceedings and more. But, in the end, if a mentally sound individual wants to refuse treatment, they have that right.

Jacob was arrested and sent to prison for the ninth time. He didn't want to be there and felt that he had received the wrong end of a short stick. He truly believed that he was being railroaded. Those pictures on his computer and the gun in his closet were not his, and he had no idea how they got there. Jacob loved to eat food and play video games and spent most days doing both. He had been placed on disabilities ten years previously. He was over 300 pounds and had no desire to change his diet, get any exercise, and he rarely left his house.

Surprisingly, when he arrived to prison, he was taking no medications. He was rather healthy, strong, and in good spirits. He had never reported depression or taken any mental health medications. These things "were not for him". The intake process and his first month in prison went by smoothly. He was happy and doing as much of the programs as possible, playing cards, getting very little exercise, and purchasing as much food from the commissary program as possible.

More than thirty days after he arrived, it became clear that he was would not be released from prison any time soon. He had been hoping to stay incarcerated for 90 days and back onto parole. The court system had different ideas. Previous sentences were enacted, and one fateful day he learned that he was going to spend five years in prison. This new information put Jacob into a tailspin. He was upset and angry. The first thing he decided to do was to begin refusing to eat.

Hunger Strikes in prison are somewhat common. Often inmates who want better meals, better living conditions, or several other things, start a hunger strike. These individuals refuse meals that come three times a day from culinary or the kitchen. Depending on the facility - a hunger strike begins after the ninth refused meal - approximately three days. Inmates also can purchase commissary and can choose several different food options. A true hunger strike occurs when they are eating nothing from commissary. Inmates are notorious for trading or maneuvering other inmates to get food. So, out of every 10 people on hunger strike, only 1 or 2 are actually not eating anything. Officers and staff try to watch closely and determine who is really refusing to eat.

Jacob was full bore, refusing to eat. On the same day he started his strike, he threw out of his cell door his entire food supply. It was quickly gathered up by other inmates. Around day five of his hunger strike, he refused to get out of bed except to go to the bathroom. Medical staff, mental health, officers, and others were coming every day or several times a day to check on him. By this point, he was refusing to talk, eat, or more. No one had observed him drinking any water. After day five, the medical staff start to get daily blood draws, vitals, and to assess him. He allowed this but refused to answer any questions.

Day after day, he would lay and sleep in the same positions, and over the next few weeks, he became less and less responsive. His vitals remained normal. After day ten or twelve, he refused to allow any additional blood tests. He would become angry if anyone came to visit him. By day seventeen, he was the talk of the entire prison. Administrators, Prison medical staff, officers, lawyers, visitors, teachers, and even the clergymen were talking about Jacob. Everybody wanted to find a way to help him, but he began refusing to allow anyone into his cell.

After three weeks, the running guess was that he had lost twenty pounds, but more concerning was that he wasn't drinking. He allowed medical into his cell every other day. His blood pressure was dropping. The medical staff didn't believe that he had gone to the bathroom in several days, and they weren't sure he was strong enough to stand on his own. A wheelchair was brought to the cell, but Jacob refused to allow it into his cell.

Jacob was never angry and never lashed out to anyone. Officers found no justification in forcing him out of his cell and into another cell. But things were rapidly getting worse. Along with not eating, Jacob hadn't showered or changed clothing. Administrators contacted local judges and other individuals to determine what they could do. A judge was contacted, and he requested to see Jacob in court. At first, Jacob agreed, likely because he thought his actions had produced enough sympathy for him to get released from prison.

The day Jacob was scheduled to go to court, he asked, "Do you know what this court thing is for?"

A newer officer responded, "They want to see if they can force you to allow an IV and force you to shower and change your clothing."

Jacob refused to go to court. By day twenty-four, things had gotten alarming. Jacob was barely awake; he was lethargic and had no energy. He couldn't lift his head off the pillow.

The medical provider came to his cell again. He asked Jacob to let him into the cell. Jacob said, "Fine."

Doctor Singh said, "Look, Jacob. Things are bad. If you lose consciousness, we will take you to the hospital. You can refuse treatment up to the point that you fall unconscious or life saving measures are required. Regardless, at this point, you are really not doing well." And not for the first time, he said, "Jacob, if you continue doing this to your body, you will die."

Jacob said, "I know. It would've been better if you guys had just released me."

"I can't control that. I'm here because your life is at risk."

Jacob began crying and said, "Take me to the hospital."

An ambulance was called. Jacob had no energy to move on his own. It took six people to transfer him onto a gurney and transport him to the waiting ambulance.

Doctor Singh noticed large stains of fluid and blood on the sheets of Jacob's bed.

When Jacob reached the hospital, they had to cut off his clothes. An IV was quickly started to give him fluids. He was dehydrated, sick, and unable to care for himself. A nasogastric (NG) tube was put into his nose to his stomach to give him some nutrition. But, by far, the worst part were the bedsores. He had spent the majority of time lying on his right side, facing the wall. He had barely moved over the last four weeks.

Bedsores are medically known as a pressure ulcer. They are common for those who lay in the same place for too long. They can be seen on diabetics, paraplegics, or even geriatrics. Often bedsores are believed to be minimally damaging. This can be true for some patients. But for those who stay in the same position for long periods of time, or have problems with healing, and especially the elderly, they can be devastating. Bedsores are categorized based on how deep they go into the skin. Early on, the sore is just redness on the skin that takes weeks to go away. Deeper tissue problems can lead to sores that go several layers into the skin. In these cases, it can appear like a hole in the skin.

Jacob had six very serious bedsores and several others. The worst sores were on his hip, lower back, leg, and ankle. But really, all his sores were significant.

The first thing the emergency room doctor asked was, "How long have you been in a wheelchair?"

Jacob answered, "Never."

"I've only seen sores like this from paraplegics that were left alone for months and months."

"I am an inmate at the prison."

The ER doctor left the exam room immediately and began berating the officer. When the officer was finally allowed to speak, he said, "The inmate did this to himself. He has been refusing food for the last 4 weeks or more. He has refused all medical care, hospital transport, or anything else the prison has tried to do."

The ER doctor replied, "I doubt that." However, when he returned to the room, Jacob confirmed that he had refused any and all treatment. But now, Jacob was worried he was going to die.

Jacob said, "Help me live."

"We will try."

Jacob had two ulcers that were large enough to fit a softball into. He spent several months at the hospital and in the medical portion of the prison. He required four surgeries to fix the damage from the ulcers. Refusing to eat had depleted his energy and the ability for his body to heal itself. His ulcers had also caused stress on his other organs. He left the hospital weighing fifty pounds less than before (or more). However, he was now diabetic, had high blood pressure, kidney problems, elevated cholesterol, neuropathy, and joint pains. It took a full year before he could walk properly again.

For the rest of his time at the prison, Jacob regretted his actions. He was trying to prove a point or get sympathy and be released. But he ended up causing himself so much more suffering and damage. He left prison and never returned again.

Made in United States
Orlando, FL
10 November 2026

90498874R00044